Praise for Taking Charge of Adult ADHD

"Powerful and essential! Your health, happiness, and future have long been a paramount concern to Dr. Barkley. Here he shares step-by-step guidance to get you where you want to be. Dr. Barkley's clear, compassionate voice makes you feel like you're in a private conversation with him. This updated second edition is worth its weight in gold."
— **Gina Pera, author of *Is It You, Me, or Adult A.D.D.?***

"This is a comprehensive and scientifically based yet comprehensible manual for understanding and managing adult ADHD. With this information, adults with ADHD or those close to them can be informed consumers of available treatment options, behavioral strategies, and supplemental support resources."
— ***Library Journal***

"Barkley knows what works."
— ***ADDitude***

"The first edition of this book was excellent; the second edition is even better! Dr. Barkley is a foremost researcher who helps you understand and cope with impairments while also developing your strengths. He provides not only practical guidance about treatment, but also strategies to avoid difficulties in education, work, relationships, money management, and health. Dr. Barkley shares his genuine empathy and personal insights into the challenges ADHD poses. This book is a valuable resource for adults with ADHD and all those who love and care for them."
— **Thomas E. Brown, PhD, author of *Smart but Stuck: Emotions in Teens and Adults with ADHD***

"The second edition of this wonderful book offers an insightful, fact-based description of how to obtain an accurate diagnosis and find appropriate help. Information is presented in a clear manner that will be helpful in guiding you through treatment. This book has earned its place as a mainstay reference."
— **Lenard A. Adler, MD, author of *Scattered Minds***

Taking Charge of Adult ADHD

Also from Russell A. Barkley

For more information, visit the author's website: *www.russellbarkley.org*

Taking Charge of Adult ADHD

Proven Strategies to Succeed at Work, at Home, and in Relationships

SECOND EDITION

Russell A. Barkley, PhD

with Christine M. Benton

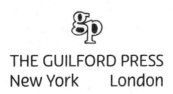

THE GUILFORD PRESS

New York   London

To my grandchildren, Will, Claire, Craig,
and Liam, the lights and loves of my life

—R. A. B.

Library of Congress Cataloging-in-Publication Data is available from the publisher.

ISBN 978-1-4625-4685-5 (paperback) — ISBN 978-1-4625-4752-4 (hardcover)

The figure on page 57 is from *12 Principles for Raising a Child with ADHD* by Russell A.
Barkley. Copyright © 2021 The Guilford Press. Reprinted by permission.

The figure on page 198 is from *ADHD in Adults: What the Science Says* by Russell A. Barkley,
Kevin R. Murphy, and Mariellen Fischer. Copyright © 2008 The Guilford Press. Reprinted
by permission.

Contents

Step Four
Change Your Life: Everyday Rules for Success

Step Five
Change Your Situation:
Mastering ADHD in Specific Areas of Your Life

• •

**Purchasers of this book can download and print enlarged
versions of the ADHD Symptom Tracking Scale
at *www.guilford.com/barkley18-forms* for personal use
or use with clients (see copyright page for details).**

• •

Acknowledgments

A number of people who assisted with the research studies that produced some of the findings in this book deserve my gratitude. First and foremost, I wish to thank Mariellen Fischer, PhD, and Kevin Murphy, PhD, for their collaboration as full partners in numerous research studies, including those made possible by three federally supported grants from the National Institute of Mental Health and the National Institute of Child Health and Human Development while I was at the University of Massachusetts Medical School. I also wish to thank Tracie Bush, Laura Montville, Lorri Bauer, Keith Douville, Cherie Horan, Hope Schrader, Kent Shiffert, and Peter Leo for their assistance in completing those sizable research studies. Furthermore, I am grateful beyond measure to the hundreds of adults with ADHD who took part in these studies and those who served in our control groups for their willingness to open their lives to us so that we could all learn more about the nature, life course, impairments, and management of ADHD in adults. Once more, I wish to extend my sincere appreciation to Kitty Moore and Seymour Weingarten at The Guilford Press for their encouragement of and assistance with this book, to Christine Benton for her insightful and constructive feedback on and sage editing of this book, and for a supportive publishing relationship with them all that has spanned more than 40 years.

Author's Note

In this book, I alternate between masculine and feminine pronouns when refer-ring to a single individual. I have made this choice to promote ease of reading as our language continues to evolve and not out of disrespect toward readers who identify with other personal pronouns. I sincerely hope that all will feel included.

All illustrations are composites of real individuals or thoroughly disguised to protect privacy.

Introduction

This book is for you if:

✓ You were diagnosed with attention-deficit/hyperactivity disorder (ADHD) as an adult.

   or

✓ You were diagnosed as a child and still have symptoms.

   or

✓ You think you might have ADHD because you have trouble . . .

  * Concentrating

  * Paying attention

  * Getting organized

  * Managing time

  * Planning and problem solving

  * Controlling your emotions

This book can help you if:

✓ You want the scientific facts about what's wrong.

✓ You want to find the best treatment.

✓ You want to learn strategies and skills to overcome your symptoms.

✓ You want to know how to play up your strengths.

ADHD is real. And it's not a condition that affects only kids. I've spent more than 40 years treating, researching, and teaching others about ADHD. For most of those years, few people believed adults could have ADHD. Now we know from closer study that as many as two-thirds of the children who have ADHD will still have it when they grow up. This means 4–5% of all adults have ADHD. **That's more than 13 million adults in the United States alone (as of 2020).**

If you're among them—or you think you might be—this book is for you. I wrote it because I think you should reap the benefits of everything we've learned from decades of research. Childhood ADHD is probably among the most extensively studied of all mental or emotional disorders. In fact, the information and advice in this book are based on *more than 400,000* research articles and books on this disorder that have been published over the last century, more than 200,000 of which were published since the last edition of this book.

We've arrived at a very good understanding of what ADHD is. We know a lot about how it affects the brain. We have a clearer view than ever of how and why the symptoms make your daily life seem like one long uphill climb.

Best of all, we have treatments that are so effective that many adults end up feeling as if the playing field has been leveled for them for the first time ever. You'll learn about them in the following pages. And based on a theory I've developed about the nature of ADHD, this book also offers you a collection of strategies that can turn your life around at work, at home, in college, and with your family and friends. These strategies are based on a scientific understanding of what's behind your symptoms, and they can help you be successful everywhere it's important to you. It's only what you deserve.

Step One
To Get Started, Get Evaluated

"Time escapes me, and I can't deal with it effectively like other adults."

"My mind and my life are a jumbled mess. I often can't seem to organize my work or other activities anywhere near as well as the other adults I know."

"I know that I flit from one thing to another and one project to another, and it drives the people I have to work with crazy. But I have to do things as soon as I think of them, because if I don't, I'll forget about them, and then they never get done."

"As a kid, I was always the one who had a hard time sitting still and had all of this energy and no clue what to do with it. I always felt like an outcast, and I hated it. I remember having to go to the nurse's office every day to take my meds—it was the worst feeling! No one wanted to be friends with me because I did not fit in with the group. I will never be the quiet, calm, reserved girl in the crowd. I am that outgoing, sometimes loud (OK, more often than I would like to admit), intense, somewhat nerdy, sarcastic, funny girl that suddenly everyone likes to be around."

"So here is what happened last weekend that my wife is so upset about. I get out the lawn mower Saturday morning to cut the grass. But the gas can is empty. So I throw it in my Ford Explorer and drive down to the Quickie Mart for gas, and while I am filling up the can, a best friend pulls in to fill up. He's as much an addict about trout fishing as I am. And he says he has an extra pole and waders, so why don't we hit the stream for a little fishing. So I say 'yeah' and get into his car and leave mine at the gas station. We fish for an hour or so, and then we're thirsty and hit this great little bar that guys love to hang out at and have a beer. It's now three in the afternoon, and I finally

3

get back to the gas station for my car, and the state police are there. You see, my wife called them when I didn't return home after several hours from getting the gas for the mower, thinking something bad had happened to me. She was so furious with me when she found out what I had done that she wouldn't talk to me for days! But that's how I am—I just go with the flow of what's happening around me and can't remember what it was I was supposed to get done, or I just blow it off as less interesting than what I might have a chance to do."

1

Is It Possible That You Have ADHD?

Do the experiences you just read about sound familiar? These are the voices of adults with ADHD. The first comment strikes at the very heart of what ADHD is. It's a succinct description of the serious time management problems that ADHD creates for adults in their daily lives. That's because adults with ADHD seem blind to time, or nearsighted toward the future. They live in the "now" and struggle to deal with all those "nexts" in life.

Do you feel like you're often out of sync with the clock, with schedules and agendas? Always late or scattered or unsure what to do with the limited hours in your day? If so, you know it's no fun feeling like you're constantly letting yourself and others down by missing deadlines and appearing to stand people up for dates and appointments. You know it's hard to maintain a sense of adult accomplishment and competence when those around you think they can't count on you to get things done or even show up. Maybe it's time to change all that.

How Would You Describe Your Problems?

Of course, time management troubles aren't caused only by ADHD. But if you share some of the other problems described by the people above, ADHD might be the culprit. And if it is, there's a lot you can do to change your life for the better.

Quickly run through this list and check off each question you'd answer with a "yes."

- ☐ Do you have trouble concentrating?

- ☐ Are you easily distracted?

- ☐ Do you consider yourself highly impulsive?

☐ Do you have trouble getting or staying organized? Do you find yourself unable to think clearly?

☐ Do you feel like you always have to be busy doing lots of things—but then you don't finish most of them?

☐ Do people say you talk too much?

☐ Is it hard for you to listen closely to others?

☐ Do you jump in and interrupt others when they're talking or doing something—and then wish you had thought first?

> You'll find a list of 91 additional symptoms associated with ADHD, gathered from a study we did over 7 years, in the Appendix (pp. 271–276).

☐ Does your voice seem to carry over everyone else's?

☐ Do you struggle to get to the point of what you're trying to say?

☐ Do you often feel restless inside?

☐ Do you find yourself forgetting things that need to get done but are not urgent?

☐ Do you find that your emotions are easily aroused and expressed, especially feeling impatient, easily frustrated, upset, or angry?

Only a professional evaluation can tell you for sure whether you have ADHD. But the more questions you answered "yes," the more likely it is that you have this disorder. What I can tell you right now is that reams of scientific data show an association between complaints like these—and hundreds of similar ones—and ADHD in adults.

The data also tell us how severe the fallout can be. ADHD can make people spend their paycheck on something fun right now—and never save enough money for their monthly or annual bill payments or for that vacation or car or house they'll want even more tomorrow than the purchase that seemed irresistible today. It can make them bet it all on an investment that a little patience and research would have revealed as a bad risk. It can make you say and do all kinds of things you later regret. And it can lead to making lots of unhealthy choices each day of your life involving impulsive eating and poor nutrition, using alcohol and tobacco, having poor sleep habits, engaging in risky sex, poor driving, and getting inadequate exercise. Sound familiar?

• • • • •

You don't have to be hyperactive to have adult ADHD.

• • • • •

But you might be thinking, I can't possibly have ADHD. I'm not hyperactive! My brother (or sister, nephew, childhood pal,

What we know about adults with ADHD comes straight from scientific fact:

- Data gathered since 1991 at the University of Massachusetts Medical School, where one of the first clinics in the United States for adults with ADHD was established, in 1990

- Evidence from a study of 158 children with ADHD (and 81 without it) followed into adulthood, one of the largest such studies done before 2010

- Even more data from numerous studies done at Massachusetts General Hospital, where another adult ADHD clinic was established around the same time as my own clinic, in 1990

- Evidence from more than 100,000 scientific articles and books on adult ADHD since the last edition of this book (2010)

classmate) had ADHD when we were kids, and he was constantly fidgety, restless, and "hyper," always acting out as if driven by a motor in some embarrassing way. *I'm not like that.*

One of the things we're beginning to understand well about adult ADHD is that hyperactivity *is* seen more in kids with the disorder—but then it usually declines substantially by adolescence and adulthood. Often the only thing that's left of hyperactivity in adults with ADHD is that feeling of restlessness and the need to keep busy that you may know well.

If you think you might have ADHD, there are good reasons to seek an evaluation:

✓ *We're coming up with lots of answers that could help you.* Adult ADHD is becoming well understood by science even though the disorder hasn't been recognized in adults for that long.

✓ *This disorder can hurt you more than a lot of other psychological problems— and it can hurt you every day, everywhere you go.* ADHD is more limiting for more patients in more areas of adult life than most other disorders seen in outpatient mental health clinics. Left untreated, it can also lead to a greater risk of mortality by midlife and a shortened overall life expectancy.

✓ *And there's a lot more help for ADHD than for a lot of other disorders that affect adults—in the form of effective treatment options and coping strategies.* ADHD is one of the most treatable psychological disorders.

How Long Have You Had These Problems?

If you think about how long you've been struggling to manage your time, to concentrate, and to control your impulses, would you say it's been just weeks or months or more like years? Picture yourself as a child: Were you dealing with any of the same problems then? Do you remember also having trouble sitting still in school? Completing your homework? Finishing a hobby project? Following the rules on a playing field? Making and keeping friends in your neighborhood? Controlling your emotions when you were frustrated or upset?

The adults with ADHD whom I've studied, diagnosed, and treated have varying memories of the types of problems you checked off earlier. Many were not diagnosed as kids. Prior to the 1980s the disorder wasn't widely recognized by clinicians. Sometimes their pediatrician didn't believe ADHD was real. Or their parents didn't think "being hyper or not being able to focus was a reason to take a child to the doctor," as one man diagnosed in his mid-20s reported. These people (and their parents!) may have bought the myth that there was nothing wrong with them that sheer willpower wouldn't cure. Sometimes people end up undiagnosed because they fall into a gray area between ADHD and non-ADHD symptoms or because they had other problems that muddied the picture.

Going undiagnosed as a child doesn't mean you don't have ADHD.

· · · · · · · ·

Having sudden, short-term symptoms usually rules out ADHD.

· · · · · · · ·

Having less severe problems managing time, concentrating, and controlling your impulses and emotions than you did as a child doesn't mean you don't have ADHD.

Being hyperactive as a child but not as an adult doesn't mean you don't have ADHD.

But not having *any* ADHD symptoms as a child or teen probably *does* mean you don't have ADHD. ADHD-like symptoms that arose only in adulthood or that haven't been going on for very long are probably being caused by something else—a brain injury or other physical illness, for example.

> Of all cases of ADHD we've diagnosed in our various clinics and studies, 98% started before age 16.

If you don't clearly remember having the same problems you just noted when you were a child, is there someone who knew you well then that you can ask? A parent? Brother or sister? Ironically, the same problems that make it hard for people with ADHD to get things done on time, make wise choices, and even get along with others can make it tough for them to trace their own history accurately—at least until they've reached approximately their mid- to late 20s. I'll explain why in Step Two.

I didn't have any problems as a child, and I haven't had any brain injuries. Isn't it possible that ADHD hasn't caused me any problems till now because of my intelligence? I scored high on IQ tests in elementary school.

Except in school and possibly at work, intelligence is unlikely to protect you from experiencing some of the impairments typically associated with ADHD, though it may have allowed you to go further in school without your ADHD being noticed than is common in typical adults who had ADHD growing up. Intelligence is not the only factor involved in domains like family and social functioning, driving, crime and drug use, dating and marital relationships, and, in fact, most others. High intelligence wouldn't necessarily have protected you in these areas if you had ADHD symptoms. The sudden appearance of problems in adulthood is highly likely to be caused by something other than ADHD.

> Children and teens with ADHD that I've followed up into adulthood often don't know the extent of their own symptoms or how much those symptoms are interfering with their life. **It's not until 27–32 years of age that adults with ADHD become more consistent in what they say about themselves relative to what others say about them.**

I think I may have ADHD now even though I didn't have any concentration or other problems when I was younger. Maybe I was just compensating for my ADHD in other ways?

In our research, the average number of major life activities in which adults with ADHD said they were often impaired was 6 or 7 out of 10. ADHD causes serious impairment across all the domains of adult life, from education to work to family. It would be nearly impossible to make it through childhood, adolescence, and even early adulthood by

• • • • • • • • • •
Symptoms must have lasted for at least 6 months to be considered in diagnosing ADHD.
• • • • • • • • • •

"compensating" somehow. Most professionals would have a hard time accepting the idea that ADHD had not interfered with a person's functioning in any major domain of life until adulthood without strong evidence that parents and schools had made extraordinary efforts to help. ADHD is defined by *lack of* compensation during the childhood years—not by successful compensation during those years!

What *Are* Your Symptoms?

Only a qualified professional can help you fully answer this question. Still, checking off any of the following questions that you'd answer "yes" will help you figure out whether to pursue a diagnostic evaluation. In our research aimed specifically at understanding adult ADHD, we've found the following nine criteria most accurate in identifying the disorder.

Do you often . . .`

☐ Get easily distracted by extraneous stimuli or irrelevant thoughts?

☐ Make decisions impulsively?

☐ Have difficulty stopping activities or behavior when you should do so?

☐ Start a project or task without reading or listening to directions carefully?

☐ Fail to follow through on promises or commitments you make to others?

☐ Have trouble doing things in their proper order or sequence?

☐ Drive much faster than others—or, if you don't drive, have difficulty engaging in leisure activities or doing fun things quietly?

> See Chapter 3 for information on finding a professional to evaluate you.

☐ Have difficulty sustaining attention in tasks or recreational activities?

☐ Have difficulty organizing tasks and activities?

Did you check off four of the first seven symptoms on the checklist, or six out of all nine symptoms? If so, you are highly likely to have ADHD. In that case you

The fifth edition of the *Diagnostic and Statistical Manual of Mental Disorders* (DSM-5), published by the American Psychiatric Association in 2013, uses 18 symptoms to diagnose ADHD—9 focusing on inattention and 9 on hyperactivity–impulsivity. But that list (see the Appendix) was initially developed for use with children only. And while this latest edition of the manual provides clarifications of some symptoms in parentheses for use with adults, those clarifications were not tested until recently, when Laura Knouse and I assessed how well they identify adults with ADHD and relate to the symptoms they clarify. We found that they were only moderately or poorly related to the original symptoms and should likely be ignored until more research is done on them.

My associates and I have also found that the checklist of nine symptoms provided above is more useful with adults than the symptom list in DSM-5. A research colleague of mine, Stephen Faraone, has done an independent study with his own groups of adults also showing that these symptoms were very good at identifying those having ADHD.

should seek an evaluation from an experienced mental health professional if you have not done so already.

How Do These Symptoms Affect Your Life?

ADHD is not a category that you either fall into or don't. It is not like pregnancy. It's more like human height or intelligence. Think of it as a dimension, with different people falling at different points along it.

> Step Five gives specific strategies for preventing ADHD symptoms from causing the impairments listed in the table.

So where on that dimension is the division between "disorder" and "no disorder"? It's where impairment in a major life activity occurs. *Symptoms* are the ways a disorder expresses itself in thoughts and actions. *Impairments* are the adverse consequences that result from showing those symptoms. The table on the next page lists typical impairments caused by ADHD in childhood and beyond.

Typical childhood impairments	Typical adolescent and adult impairments
Family stress and conflict	Poor functioning at work
Poor peer relationships	Frequent job changes
Few or no close friendships	Risky sexual behavior/increased teen pregnancy and sexually transmitted diseases
Disruptive behavior in stores, church, and other community settings to the extent that you are asked to leave or not return	Difficulties managing anger and frustration in intimate relationships
Low regard for personal safety/ increased accidental injuries	Unsafe driving (speeding, frequent accidents, numerous parking violations, possible license suspension)
Slow development of self-care	Difficulties managing finances (impulsive spending, excessive use of credit cards, poor debt repayment, little or no savings, and so on)
Slow development of personal responsibility	Problems in dating or marital relationships (don't seem to listen to or appreciate the needs of your partner, talk excessively and interrupt, fail to follow through on promises and commitments)
Significantly lower than average school performance	Prone to excessive use of substances such as tobacco, alcohol, or marijuana
Significantly fewer years of schooling	Difficulty getting to sleep at a reasonable hour (insomnia), frequent night waking and restlessness, inefficient sleep leading to daytime tiredness
	Less common but notable:
	Antisocial activities (lying, stealing, fighting) that lead to frequent police contact, arrests, and even jail time; often associated with a greater risk for illegal drug use and abuse
	Generally less healthy lifestyle (less exercise; more sedentary self-entertainment, such as video games, TV, surfing the Internet; greater use of social media; obesity, binge eating or bulimia, poorer nutrition; greater use of nicotine and alcohol); consequently increased risk for later coronary heart disease

What's Next?

Now you should have a fairly good idea of whether you might have ADHD and should consider a professional evaluation:

- ☐ Do you have at least four to six of the nine symptoms now?

- ☐ Do they occur often in your current life?

- ☐ Have you been having these troubles for at least 6 months?

- ☐ Did they develop in childhood or adolescence (before 16 years of age)?

- ☐ Have your current symptoms resulted in adverse consequences (impairment) in one or more major domains (such as education, work, social relationships, dating or marital relationships, managing your money, driving)?

- ☐ Did you experience adverse consequences from these symptoms in childhood?

If you can answer "yes" to all of these questions, there is a high probability that you have ADHD. Read on to find out what you can do about it.

2

Can You Handle
the Problem
on Your Own?

Believing you might have ADHD can feel like a huge relief: At last you have some idea of why your life has been so tough. Problem solved, right? All you have to do now is read a couple books like this one so you know how to deal with the deficits ADHD imposes.

Not so fast. There are some very powerful reasons to get professional help, both for diagnosis and for treatment. This chapter will explain in more depth what one man in his 30s put so plainly:

> "I've tried extremely hard over the past few decades to deal with my ADHD on my own and feel I've done OK. But now I think I need some help. I'm tired of being a 'skipping stone' as far as careers go and would really like to settle and excel as I KNOW I can."

In brief, these are the reasons to get professional help:

✓ To make sure your symptoms aren't being caused by a condition other than ADHD that requires attention

✓ To discover whether your problems are being caused by a combination of ADHD and another condition

✓ To get the prescription medication that's proven to give a huge boost to coping efforts if you do receive a diagnosis of ADHD

✓ To gain access to the latest psychological therapies that can address your various problems with self-control

✓ To find out where your strengths and weaknesses are so you can aim your coping efforts exactly where they're needed

✓ To get an evaluation that can serve as the basis for getting appropriate accommodations in college, other educational settings, or the workplace under the Americans with Disabilities Act

✓ To access other resources that may help you change an unhealthy lifestyle and poor health maintenance practices, such as assistance with weight loss, quitting smoking, reducing alcohol or marijuana use, or improving your sleep

All great reasons to form a relationship with a doctor who can prescribe the right treatment for you and get you access to various services, protections, and entitlements.

Convinced? If so, feel free to turn directly to Chapter 3. But if you need to know more about why you should not try to handle this problem alone, read the rest of this chapter.

Are Your Symptoms Being Caused by Something Else, Like a Medical Problem?

Let's go back to the idea that knowing you might have ADHD can be a relief. We've found that finding a name and a neurobiological reason for many of your struggles is, in itself, therapeutic. When you know what's wrong, you can stop beating yourself up for not being able to just shake off your problems. But you can't truly *know* you have ADHD without that evaluation. Only a seasoned mental health professional has the training and judgment to apply the diagnostic criteria you learned about in Chapter 1. Without that kind of background, you won't be able to factor in the nuances that define the line between signs of ADHD and symptoms that can be found to lesser degrees in the general population of adults. Nor will you be familiar with the other psychological and psychiatric disorders that cause problems with attention, concentration, and working memory so that you can distinguish between those and ADHD.

Just as important, a qualified professional can direct you to any medical tests or procedures you need to ensure that your symptoms are not a result of brain injury or illness, as noted in Chapter 1.

> Wouldn't it be an even bigger relief to *know* you have ADHD than to just *guess*?

Does ADHD Explain Everything You're Going Through?

Even if Chapter 1 gave you a strong feeling that you have ADHD, you need a professional evaluation to make sure ADHD tells the whole story. It would be incredibly demoralizing to address ADHD and still struggle because some other problem has gone undiscovered and untreated. If an evaluation turns up coexisting disorders (called *comorbidity*), you'll be given not only a diagnosis and some information about your disorder(s) but also a list of treatment recommendations—the first step on your way to leaving behind your life as a "skipping stone."

> Most adults with ADHD who are seen in clinics have at least two disorders: 80–85% have ADHD and one other disorder, and more than half may have three psychological disorders.

Other Disorders That Co-Occur More Often in Those with ADHD Than in the General Population

Anxiety disorders

Oppositional defiant disorder (ODD)

Conduct disorder (CD; aggression, delinquency, truancy, and the like)

Learning disabilities (LDs; delays in areas like reading, spelling, math, writing)

Demoralization, dysthymia, or outright major depression

Childhood- or adolescent-onset bipolar disorder

Adult antisocial personality disorder (ASPD)

Alcoholism and other addictions

Tic disorders or the more severe Tourette syndrome (multiple motor and vocal tics)

Autism spectrum disorders

The Most Effective Treatment—Medication— Requires a Doctor's Prescription

• • • • • • • •

The success rate for ADHD medications is probably unrivaled by any other medication treatment for any other disorder in psychiatry.

• • • • • • • •

You can read all about the medications used to treat ADHD in Step Three. What's important to know right now is that where ADHD symptoms are concerned, *medication works.* It improves the symptoms, often substantially. It is effective in a large percentage of adults—fewer than 10% will have *no* positive response to any of the drugs approved for use with ADHD. Medication even seems to temporarily correct or compensate for the underlying neurological problems that are likely contributing to the ADHD in the first place.

A lot of other treatments and coping methods have little effect *unless* the person with ADHD is also taking medication. In my experience, adults with ADHD who choose not to try medication following their diagnosis typically return within 3–6 months asking to go on it once they realize that all the other options are not addressing their problems very well.

Studies show that ADHD medications can:

- *Normalize* the behavior of 50–65% of those with ADHD

- *Substantially improve* the behavior of another 20–30% of people with the disorder

Exactly What Are Your Strengths and Weaknesses?

A professional evaluation involves several steps. These steps are designed to look at your difficulties from a number of angles to make sure important facts aren't overlooked or signs misinterpreted. But if the process seems repetitive or drawn out to you, keep in mind that the evaluator is trying to rule out things that are *not* causing you problems as well as identify what *is* causing you trouble. There's another reason to be patient with this process: In differentiating among all the possible causes of your symptoms, the practitioner will also be unearthing valuable information about your personal strengths. Knowing where you shine in life skills and natural abilities will help you and your therapist choose coping strategies that are tailored to help you most. Artistic talents and engaging personalities, for instance, don't come from having ADHD, but you can learn to use these gifts to compensate for ADHD symptoms. Or you can identify a career path that draws on these strengths.

I've met many representatives for pharmaceutical companies, for example, who have ADHD but are outstanding in their work. The job allows them to travel extensively and meet with lots of different physicians and their office staff, keeping them engaged and on the go. A nine-to-five desk job might prove so boring that they would be hard-pressed to concentrate and stay motivated to succeed despite their natural talent for salesmanship and customer relations. But the constant change of scene energizes and focuses these reps. Many also work in teams with other reps to cover a region, which gives their work some structure that would not be available to them in a solo sales position.

That's what the evaluation process is all about: finding out exactly what's wrong and what you have going for you so that a treatment plan can be designed to set you on the road to health and success as quickly as possible.

3

Where Can You Go to Get Help?

If you haven't yet had a diagnostic evaluation, you can seek a qualified mental health professional on your own. But if you have a good relationship with your primary care physician, a call to this doctor might be a fruitful first step. A doctor who knows you well can use screening questionnaires to determine whether you're right to think you could have ADHD. If the doctor can rule out physical causes for your symptoms, you've spared yourself the separate medical exam that a mental health evaluator might recommend. And a physician who knows you well may be able to refer you to an ADHD specialist who is likely to be a good fit for you. In my experience, when you like and trust your doctor, you have a good chance of feeling the same way about anyone the doctor recommends.

How to Find a Professional Who Is Experienced with ADHD

Any of the following could be a good source of referrals. If one doesn't pan out for you, try one of the others.

✔ As mentioned above, you might start by calling your primary care provider (internist, family practitioner, or general practitioner) to ask for the name of a specialist in your area who is working in adult ADHD.

✔ Call your state psychiatric association or psychological association. The state associations usually keep lists of their professionals, organized by specialty. See if they have any who are listed as experts focusing on ADHD in adults.

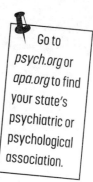
Go to *psych.org* or *apa.org* to find your state's psychiatric or psychological association.

✓ Check the website of one of the major nonprofit organizations dedicated to ADHD: CHADD (United States) and ADDA (United States and other English-speaking countries). If either one has a support group or chapter in your area, call and ask if they know of any adult ADHD clinical experts in your area.

✓ Call the local university medical school psychiatry department. Even if it's not nearby, they can usually direct you to the practitioners they know in your area who do adult ADHD evaluations. Or go to their website to see if ADHD is listed as one of the disorders in which they specialize.

> Website for Children and Adults with Attention-Deficit/Hyperactivity Disorder (CHADD): *chadd.org.*
>
> Website for the Attention Deficit Disorder Association (ADDA): *add.org.*
>
> Other websites that can be useful in finding professionals specializing in adult ADHD can be found in the Resources at the back of the book.

✓ Call the local hospital psychiatry department for the same information. Or, again, go to their website to see if ADHD is listed as one of the disorders in which they specialize.

✓ Call the local university psychology clinic for the same information. Or go to their website to see if ADHD is listed as one of the disorders in which they specialize.

✓ Call the county mental health center (usually listed in your phone book under "county government"). Or go to their website to see if ADHD is listed as one of the disorders in which they specialize.

✓ Check the yellow pages for psychiatrists and psychologists specializing in adult ADHD. Or, better yet, go online and search for ADHD professionals in your city or state. Physicians and psychiatrists can also specifically search their region for such professionals. Also both *chadd.org* and *additudemag.com* provide options to search for ADHD professionals in your area.

✓ Do you have a friend or relative you trust who is being treated for adult ADHD? If so, ask for a referral to that person's practitioner. Or if you know someone whose child is being treated for ADHD, you might ask for the child's doctor's name and call that clinician to see if he or she treats adults or knows someone who does.

Questions to Ask before You Make an Appointment

If you're lucky enough to have a number of specialists to choose from in your area, you can ask the following questions when you call to inquire about an evaluation. In fact, you might want to ask these questions even if you've located only one professional nearby:

✓ What percentage of the doctor's practice is made up of people with ADHD (as opposed to other disorders)?

✓ If the practitioner sees both adults and children, what percentage are adults?

✓ How long has the doctor been treating adults with ADHD?

✓ What is the practitioner's area of specialization in medicine or psychology? Fields that cover ADHD and related psychiatric disorders include psychiatry, clinical psychology, neuropsychology, and neurology (especially behavioral).

✓ Is the practitioner board certified in this area of specialization? Board certification is a higher level of certification than a state license to practice medicine or psychology.

✓ How long will it take to get an appointment? (This may be significant to you if you have a number of professionals to choose from and would like to be seen as soon as possible.)

✓ Does the doctor treat people after diagnosing them? If not, where are patients referred for treatment?

✓ Are other potential resources available nearby? Most mental health practitioners will not have coaching, skills training, support groups, and the like on site, but psychologists in private practice often rent space in office parks where related professionals work, and they all refer patients to each other.

✓ How does the doctor charge, and what insurance plans does he or she accept?

4

What Do You Need for the Evaluation?

When you know what to expect, the evaluation process is likely to proceed more smoothly and quickly.

Prepare by Knowing What to Expect and What to Take Along

Here are the typical elements in a diagnostic evaluation:

✓ Collection of rating scales and referral information before or during the evaluation

✓ An interview with you

✓ A review of previous records that may document your impairments

✓ Psychological testing to rule out general cognitive delay or LDs

✓ Interviews with others who know you well to corroborate your reports

✓ A general medical examination when medication might be part of your treatment or coexisting medical conditions need to be evaluated (if your physician hasn't already done this)

What you can take along to facilitate these steps:

✓ Any records you have or can collect in advance from schools you attended and physicians and mental health professionals you've seen, any driving and criminal records, and any other documentation of problems that could be related to ADHD or another disorder

✓ The names of a few people who know you well and whom you trust to speak honestly and objectively with the evaluators

✓ Results of a medical exam if you've already had one from your physician

✓ A list of family members with mental disorders you know about

✓ A description of impairments during childhood and adolescence, as well as more recent ones

Take Along an Open Mind

You've made this appointment because you want answers: Why can't you get done what adults need to do? Why do you keep struggling despite huge efforts to "buckle down" and succeed? What will it take for you to be able to reach important personal and professional goals? To provide these answers, the clinician you've made an appointment with has to gather a lot of information from a lot of sources. You may question the need for all of it. You might feel restless in the middle of the evaluation, eager to get it over with. Try to stay focused on the goal—answers and solutions—and remember that the most important thing to take to your evaluation appointment is **an open mind.**

> **Be prepared** for the initial evaluation appointment to take several hours.

Go along with requests for school and other records, even though your academic history may be the last thing you want to revisit. Answer questions about impairment as honestly as you can. Be open to letting the evaluator interview someone else who knows you well to get a helpful outside perspective. Every test, questionnaire, and interview included in the evaluation has a scientific basis and is designed to provide the most reliable answers that the field of psychology can deliver.

With all these tests, rating scales, questionnaires, past records, and interviews, the psychologist knows everything there is to know about me. Why does she need to talk to one of my relatives too?

The short answer is that there's strength in numbers. The more different sources the evaluator can use to confirm your symptoms and the impairment you've suffered, the firmer the conclusions that can be drawn. That's why the evaluator doesn't just talk to you; she also uses scientifically devised rating scales and other tools to come at the information from as many angles as possible.

But even with all these tools, the evaluator is getting all the input from you. The fact is that adults (and children) with ADHD often report doing better on certain tasks than outside observation and objective measurements reveal. Driving is a particularly common example. You may very well believe you're just as good a driver as anyone else (or even better than average). You might feel those speeding tickets you've piled up were unfair, written by a police officer who was prejudiced against you or just trying to fill his quota for the month. Fender benders you've had may seem like they were caused by the other driver, who wasn't paying enough attention or who was too hesitant and therefore sent you misleading signals. And all those parking tickets because you just didn't have time to find a legal spot—well, everyone gets those, don't they? Someone who knows you well and—this is essential—is in your corner and wants to help you, not just criticize you, might be able to say that in fact you do drive much faster than most people, that your attention sometimes drifts from the road, that you try to multitask or text message while driving, and that you get impatient easily when traffic backs up. On the surface it may feel like an intrusion but try to believe that it is in your own best interest to let the professional speak about your concerns and your history with someone who knows you well, such as a parent, sibling, spouse or live-in partner, or close friend if family members are not available. Without this perspective, it might appear that you do not have ADHD when in fact you actually do have it, given the information that others can provide about you. Keep in mind that you're here to get answers—and accurate ones.

 Why in the world would it matter that Aunt Ellen spent most of her life depressed? What does that have to do with me?

Heredity (genes) contributes to most mental disorders to varying degrees. This means that relatives of people with mental disorders are more likely to develop the same disorders. The types of disorders seen in your relatives can serve as a guide to the sorts of disorders you may be experiencing. ADHD is a highly genetic disorder, more so than most in psychiatry, so unless you have acquired it through an obvious brain injury in your past, it's likely to be more common than usual among your relatives. But because adults with ADHD frequently have another disorder too (see Chapter 2), it can be helpful to the evaluator to know about all mental disorders that appear on your family tree and for which you may have a genetic vulnerability. If you're not aware of any, that may be because in the past people tended to view such information as private, even shameful. For this reason, it's worth taking the trouble to ask a parent or other relative from a generation before yours about the history of mental disorders in your family before you go to your appointment.

Stay Focused on Getting Answers

Test taking may not hold great memories for you. But try to remember during the string of psychological tests usually given that you and the evaluator share the same goal: to get answers. You wouldn't want those answers to be based on opinion alone, so do your best to take these tests openly and honestly. On the other hand, don't let anyone tell you that the results of any one test are a foolproof indication that you do or do not have ADHD. There is no diagnostic test for ADHD that is accurate enough to be used in clinical practice. Diagnosis is an art as well as a science. Accurate diagnosis depends on the adept analysis of a professional with the experience to weigh the results gained from different sources and different parts of the evaluation. This is the best way to get an accurate picture of your problem.

Psychological Tests Typically Given during an Evaluation

✓ *Brief test of your intelligence or general cognitive ability:* Sometimes people struggle in school or at work because of limitations in their intellectual or learning abilities. The professional needs to rule out these types of limitations as a cause of or contributor to your ADHD-like symptoms or their impact on your educational and work difficulties.

> *From 35 to 85% of people with ADHD can pass tests of attention, inhibition, and working memory and yet still have the disorder.* Researchers have found that if people do poorly on these sorts of tests, they probably do have some sort of disorder. That does not mean that it is ADHD, however, because other disorders can interfere with performing these tests normally. On the other hand, getting normal scores on these tests does not mean the professional can rule out ADHD.

✓ *Tests involving reading, math, and spelling:* These are especially likely to be given if you are in an educational setting, like college, technical training, or work-related education. People with ADHD are far more likely than others to also have specific delays in academic abilities such as these, often called *specific learning disabilities,* and it's important to know if you have them.

✓ *Tests of attention, inhibition, and memory:* Not all psychologists give these tests. I don't recommend their use for diagnosing ADHD as they are not sufficiently accurate. The significance of the results can be exaggerated if it's assumed they are objective measures of ADHD and therefore more reliable than your own oral reports of symptoms and the data from other parts of the evaluation. Abnormal scores can indicate ADHD or other disorders—but that doesn't mean that normal scores alone rule out ADHD.

5

What Will the Evaluation Tell You?

In most cases you'll get the answers you came for on the spot, in a feedback conference that concludes the evaluation. In a few instances, if the results of any testing done are not immediately available, the feedback conference may be delayed. During the conference the professional will:

✓ Discuss the findings from all the information gathering

✓ Give you an opinion about whether you have ADHD or other problems

✓ Provide a set of recommendations for what to do about your ADHD and any other problems uncovered

To render a diagnosis of adult ADHD, the professional must believe from the evaluation's findings that:

✓ You have high levels of inattention and/or hyperactive and impulsive behavior

✓ You have these symptoms far more often than other adults your age

✓ You've had these symptoms, in their current form, for at least 6 months

✓ Your symptoms developed before you were 12–16 years old

> It's possible to have ADHD without having problems with impulsivity or hyperactivity. There's a "presentation" of ADHD characterized mainly by problems with inattention. (More on this presentation on pages 35–36.)

✓ Your symptoms have had adverse consequences for you in many different domains in both your childhood and your adult life

As my colleague Kevin Murphy, PhD, has written, your evaluation for ADHD should be designed to answer four fundamental questions:

1. Is there credible evidence that you experienced ADHD-type symptoms in early childhood that, at least by the middle school years, led to substantial and chronic impairment across settings?

2. Is there credible evidence that ADHD-type symptoms currently cause you substantial and consistent impairment across settings?

3. Are there explanations other than ADHD that better account for your array of current concerns?

4. If you meet the criteria for ADHD, is there evidence that you have any other disorders as well?

Do Your Symptoms Meet the Criteria for ADHD?

First and foremost, the evaluator will compare what he or she has learned about your symptoms with the criteria for diagnosing ADHD listed in the latest edition of the American Psychiatric Association's DSM. According to the DSM, to be diagnosed with ADHD, you are supposed to have at least five of the symptoms included in either of the two nine-item lists—one centering on inattention and the other on hyperactivity–impulsivity—mentioned in Chapter 1 and shown in the Appendix. There are two problems with this guideline:

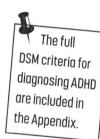 The full DSM criteria for diagnosing ADHD are included in the Appendix.

If the evaluator says you don't have ADHD because you have fewer than the five DSM criteria, indicate that my research and that of others has shown just four symptoms is enough to be considered clinically significant. Or ask to be evaluated again using our nine-item list (page 10).

1. Lots of research has shown that many people do have all the earmarks of ADHD *without* having the full five symptoms from either symptom list. Several studies, my own included, have shown that you actually need only four of the symptoms on either list to be having these problems to a degree inappropriate for an adult.

2. These criteria were originally designed to diagnose children, not adults (which I am well aware of since I was a member of the committee that established them).

This is why my colleagues and I rely on the nine-criteria list you've already read on page 10 as much as or more than the DSM-5 symptoms. It is based on everything research has revealed about *adults* with ADHD and has already proven effective in accurately diagnosing hundreds of adults in the 12 years since we first identified this set of items as useful.

Essentially, the evaluation will translate your personal experiences into criteria designed to separate those with ADHD from those without ADHD so you can receive whatever help you need—and avoid being treated for a disorder you *don't* have.

We used a variety of statistical methods to identify the symptoms that are most essential in distinguishing the adults with ADHD. In doing so we compared them not only to the community ("typical") adults but to a second control group of adults seen at the same mental health clinic who had other psychological disorders but did not have ADHD. We also added into our analyses the 18 items from the DSM to see just how good they were at identifying ADHD in adults.

We found that, surprisingly, just nine of the 109 symptoms we identified (see the Appendix) are needed to identify adults with ADHD—the nine you've already seen in Chapter 1.

Does the Diagnosis Sound Like You?

Let's take a closer look at those abstract-sounding symptoms. ADHD basically consists of problems in three separate areas that you may experience in these ways:

✓ *Short attention span or lack of persistence on tasks:* You may notice this group of symptoms particularly when you are expected to do something tedious, boring, or drawn out.

- Do you quickly get bored during repetitive tasks?

- Do you shift from one uncompleted activity to another (say, with housecleaning, half making the bed and then emptying part of the dishwasher and then dusting only one room)?

- Do you lose your concentration during a long task, finding it almost impossible to write an in-depth report or fill out a tax return with its many schedules and forms?

- Do you have a hard time getting in your sales or other status reports on time without being "nagged" by your boss?

Many people with ADHD describe a double whammy in this area: They can't seem to concentrate long enough to finish routine tasks, and they're also distracted by virtually anything else that enters their field of consciousness. Someone enters their peripheral vision, their eye follows, and their mind goes along for the ride, never to return from its detour. Or unbidden and unwelcome irrelevant thoughts suddenly pop into their head, and their mind wanders off on a tangent that takes them so far off course that they lose tons of time.

✔ *Impaired ability to control impulses and delay gratification:*

- Do people criticize you for not "looking before you leap"?

- Is "What were you *thinking?*" a question you hear at least a couple times a week because of something you said or did without much regard for the consequences?

- Have you embarrassed yourself by interrupting others, blurting out comments you wish you had bitten back, or dominating the conversation until everyone else leaves in disgust?

- Do you put off necessary errands when there's a line at the bank, the post office, or the supermarket checkout?

- Do you always have a second piece of cake or other fattening food even though you really want to lose 10 pounds?

- Do you spend your paycheck every weekend instead of saving for the ski equipment or some other large item that you want or need?

Many teens and adults with ADHD tend to speed when they drive, to lose patience with other drivers and drive aggressively, to rack up parking tickets because they just can't be bothered to find a legal parking space, and generally to have a very low tolerance for frustration. Is this you?

✓ *Excessive or uncontrolled activity or activity that's irrelevant to the task at hand:* Most—but not all—adults with ADHD were fidgety, restless, and "on the go" as children.

- Do you remember moving in ways that weren't needed to complete the task you were assigned, such as wriggling your feet and legs, squirming in your seat, tapping your hands or feet, touching things frequently, rocking, or often shifting your position while performing relatively boring tasks?

If this was part of your childhood experience, you may be aware that it's changed as you've matured: maybe now you would describe yourself as restless, antsy, always needing to be busy.

How Are Those Symptoms Really Affecting Your Life?

Symptoms alone aren't enough to produce a diagnosis of ADHD. You have to be *impaired* by those symptoms.

Impairment = the social and other adverse consequences or costs that result from expressing the symptoms of ADHD.

But there's another element to the term that's just as important as this definition: Impairment is defined relative to the average person in the population, known as the *norm*—it is where most "normal," or typical, people are found to be performing in any domain of life. It does not mean how you are functioning compared to incredibly bright or highly educated people even if you are one. To be impaired, you must be functioning significantly below the norm or the average (typical) person. Why? Because the term *disorder* means just that—you are not functioning typically.

Earlier I called impairment the *adverse consequences* that can result from your behavior or symptoms. They involve the environment kicking back, so to speak, as a result of your displaying such behavior. These can involve just about anything that can be negatively affected in your life. If you look at the 91 symptoms listed in the Appendix, it will give you an idea of how many different ways ADHD could be expressing itself in your life. I suspect you already know what the adverse consequences of those symptoms can be.

ADHD symptoms can cause impairments in every domain of your life:

Home   Work   Social life   Community   Education

Dating/marriage   Money management   Driving   Leisure activities

Sexual behavior   Child rearing   Daily responsibilities

Having trouble resisting impulses might lead to extramarital affairs and consequently divorce. It might make you buy things you can't afford but think you can't live without at the moment. It could lead you to abandon simple obligations like child care or personal hygiene. Difficulty taking constructive criticism and making changes based on feedback from authority figures can leave you stalled in your career (or fired) and getting less out of educational opportunities than you could. Having a poor grasp of time can leave you missing important appointments and celebrations, compromising your personal as well as professional relationships. Problems with memory, reading comprehension, and mental arithmetic can make even the most basic daily tasks a frustrating challenge to complete. Overreacting emotionally can cause problems in every arena of your life, robbing you of chances to contribute to your community through civic or volunteer work, making you susceptible to road rage, and potentially costing you jobs, friends, and more intimate relationships. These are just a few examples of the damage that ADHD symptoms can do.

Can You Accept the Professional's Conclusions?

We're all human, and part of being human is going into certain situations with our minds made up—or at least with a healthy dose of skepticism. If you approached the evaluation with a strong opinion about whether you do or do not have ADHD, that opinion could very well color your reaction to the professional's feedback. Here are a few things to think about before rejecting the opinion of the professionals you're consulting:

The "Everyone Has ADHD Symptoms" Myth

That ADHD is a legitimate, real disorder has been questioned repeatedly over the years. Naysayers argue that typical individuals in the general population have the same kinds of symptoms and impairments that supposedly exist only in those diagnosed with the disorder. It's true that people who would be considered the norm may show some of the behavioral characteristics of ADHD *once in a while.* Everyone feels particularly distractible on some days or has trouble concentrating on others. What distinguishes adults with ADHD from others is the considerably greater frequency with which they display these characteristics. Distractibility, inability to concentrate, and other problems reach a point of being developmentally inappropriate (rare) for their age group.

My colleagues and I published a book in 2008 containing a study in which we asked 146 adults diagnosed with ADHD and 109 adults from a general community sample to tell us whether they had experienced the 18 DSM symptoms *often.* The answers are shown in the table on the facing page.

Adults with ADHD versus typical adults:

- Fewer than 10% of the typical adults answered "yes" to all but two of these questions.

- 12% or fewer did so for the other two questions.

- On average, adults in the general-population control group reported less than 1 symptom out of all 18, whereas adults with ADHD reported more than 12 (7 on the inattention list and 5 on the hyperactive–impulsive list).

Clearly the vast majority of typical adults do not report having these problems often. There is a quantifiable, statistically significant, and noticeable difference between the experiences of those diagnosed with ADHD and others.

In the same study, we asked adults with ADHD and those in the community population in what domains of life they were often *impaired* by ADHD symptoms. The results we got are in the table on page 34.

For every one of these major life activities more of the adults with ADHD reported being impaired than did the adults in the general population. In most areas, a substantial majority reported that they were "often" impaired.

The same people who claim that so-called ADHD symptoms are problems

Symptom	Adults with ADHD (%)	Adults in the community (%)
Inattention symptoms		
Fails to give close attention to details	74	3
Difficulty sustaining attention	97	3
Fails to listen when spoken to directly	73	2
Doesn't follow through on instructions	75	1
Has difficulty organizing tasks	81	5
Avoids tasks requiring sustained mental effort	81	2
Loses necessary things	75	11
Easily distracted by extraneous stimuli	97	2
Forgetful in daily activities	78	4
Hyperactive–impulsive symptoms		
Fidgets with hand/feet or squirms in seat	79	4
Leaves seat when required to stay seated	30	2
Feels restless	77	3
Difficulty doing leisure activities quietly	38	3
Has to be "on the go"	62	12
Talks excessively	44	4
Blurts out answers	57	7
Difficulty awaiting turn	67	3
Interrupts or intrudes on others	57	3

that all adults have often claim that these symptoms (and impairments) are even more pronounced and prevalent in "typical" children than "typical" adults. ADHD is not a disorder, they say, but just a set of problems widely experienced by the general population, especially in childhood. Not so, our study showed.

You can find the results of our studies comparing symptoms and domains where impairments occurred in *children* with and without ADHD in a book I wrote with Kevin Murphy and Mariellen Fischer, *ADHD in Adults: What the Science Says* (Guilford Press, 2008). The table of 91 symptoms in the Appendix also shows a huge disparity between adults with and without ADHD.

Domain of life	Adults with ADHD (%)	Adults in the community (%)
Home life	69	2
Work or occupation	75	2
Social interactions	56	1
Community activities	44	1
Educational activities	89	1
Dating or marital activities	73	1
Money management	73	1
Driving	38	2
Leisure activities	46	1
Daily responsibilities	86	2

When You Don't Quite Fit the Picture of ADHD

The professional who evaluates you may tell you that you seem to have a particular "presentation" of ADHD but that he or she is not sure. Currently, DSM-5 divides ADHD into three presentations:

1. Predominantly hyperactive

2. Predominantly inattentive

3. Combined

The trouble is, this subdivision sometimes muddies the diagnostic waters because the groups overlap and may represent a range of severity rather than three distinct types, and people can move across these presentations, just as a function of time. So don't view these presentations as being somehow qualitatively different forms of the disorder that are stable over time—they are not.

To confuse matters further, 30–50% of those who seem to have the predominantly inattentive presentation of ADHD may not have ADHD at all but something that some researchers, including me, now call a "sluggish cognitive tempo" (SCT), a separate deficiency in a different type of attention.

Do you think you might have the following tendencies, some of which seem like the *opposite* of ADHD?

☐ Daydreaming

☐ Being spacey

☐ Staring frequently

☐ Being slow moving, hypoactive, lethargic, and sluggish

☐ Being easily confused or mentally "foggy"

☐ Being slow to process information and prone to making mistakes in doing so

☐ Having a poor focus of attention or being unable to distinguish what is important from what is not in information that has to be processed quickly

The three presentations of ADHD as of 2013:

- The *combined presentation* is the most common (approximately 65% or more of clinical cases) and the most severe and involves 10 or more of all the characteristics noted in the 18 DSM criteria (5+ for inattention and 5+ for hyperactive–impulsive). It's also the most extensively studied of the "types" of ADHD, with thousands of scientific studies on this group published over the last 100 years.

- The *predominantly hyperactive presentation* was recognized in 1994. People with this type of ADHD don't have sufficient problems with inattentiveness to be diagnosed with the combined type. It shows up mainly as difficulties with impulsive and hyperactive behavior and is most often seen in preschool children, even before their inattention becomes obvious. It's now believed to represent simply an early developmental stage of the combined presentation in most cases. As many as 90% of these people will develop enough problems with attention and distractibility to be diagnosed eventually with the combined presentation within 3–5 years. The remaining cases appear to mostly represent a milder variant of the combined presentation.

- Individuals who exhibit chiefly attention problems but not excessive activity levels or poor impulse control are considered to have the *predominantly inattentive presentation* of ADHD. First recognized around 1980, this subgroup makes up about 30% or more of clinically referred cases. Many of these cases are just milder forms of the combined presentation.

☐ Having more problems consistently remembering information that was previously learned

☐ Being more socially reticent, shy, or withdrawn than others

☐ Being more passive or even hesitant instead of being impulsive (like the more typical combined type of ADHD)

☐ Having a pattern of comorbid disorders that differs from that commonly seen in ADHD, such as:

  ☐ Rarely showing social aggression (ODD)

  ☐ Less likely to be antisocial or have CD (frequent lying, stealing, fighting, and so forth)

  ☐ More likely to be depressed and possibly anxious

  ☐ LDs or impaired schoolwork due to making errors rather than reduced productivity or disruptive class behavior

If this pattern seems like it might fit you, ask the professional who evaluated you. So little is known scientifically about this syndrome that it won't be discussed further in this book. See the Fact Sheets page on my website (*russellbarkley.org*) for more information.

What If You Still
Disagree with the Professional's Conclusions?

You've now read all about ADHD and how it's diagnosed. Maybe you've received a diagnosis yourself. Are you ready to own this disorder? It's the only way to seek appropriate treatment and get on with the kind of life you want and deserve.

When Is a Second Opinion Warranted?

If you find yourself disagreeing with the results of your first evaluation, ask yourself honestly whether you disagree because your professional did such a poor or cursory job evaluating you or concluded things about your behavior that you know are simply not true. If so, you should seek a second opinion.

But even if the evaluation was done responsibly and well, and the feedback you were given sounds like it describes you, you may disagree with the label. The problem may be your preconceived notions or your own attempts at self-diagnosis. Sometimes people seek professional evaluations believing they have a particular disorder, such as bipolar disorder, only to be told by the professional that what they really have is ADHD. When the professional's diagnosis conflicts with what they originally believed, it can be hard to accept. In a case like this, you can surely seek a second opinion. But know that you're not likely to be satisfied with that one either, because it will again disagree with your self-diagnosis. Second opinions are reasonable to pursue as long as you have solid, rational grounds on which to question the initial evaluation and disagree with its conclusions.

If you're tempted to seek a second opinion because you think you *do* have ADHD but the professional says you don't, see the sidebar on pages 38–39.

A Final Reality Check

If you've received a diagnosis of ADHD but are not quite ready to own the disorder, take a look at these fast facts. You're not alone:

- ✓ ADHD occurs in approximately 5–8% of the childhood population and 4–5% of adults, or as many as 13.6 million as of 2020.

- ✓ In childhood it is three times more common in boys than girls, but by adulthood the ratio of males to females is approximately 1.6 to 1 or less.

- ✓ The disorder is found in all countries and ethnic groups studied to date.

- ✓ ADHD is somewhat more common in urban and population-dense regions than in suburban or rural settings and is found across all social classes.

- ✓ ADHD is more common among people in certain professions, such as the military, the trades, the performing arts, and sales, and among professional athletes, physical education teachers, and entrepreneurs, than among those in other fields.

Being among this group is not necessarily devastating news. There's a lot of help available. But that help requires that you acknowledge, accept, and own the diagnosis of ADHD as being a part of who you are. Otherwise, you will be far less committed to seeking appropriate treatment or to following through on the advice you get from professionals.

Ready to start getting that help?

What If the Professional Says You Don't Have ADHD but You Believe You Do?

There's a funny thing about ADHD: perhaps because its impact on achievement is so well known, many people blame the disorder when they don't meet their own standards for accomplishment. Do any of these people sound like you?

Joe decided to become a doctor when he was in high school. So he chose a college with a great biology department and a high rate of admission to medical schools. He got into that university only on the waiting list, but at least he got in. Once he was there, though, every science course was a struggle for him. By junior year his GPA was hovering under a 3.0, and he had already taken organic chemistry three times without passing. Joe started to wonder what in the world was wrong with him: he worked so hard, he wanted this so badly, and he was just as intelligent as the next guy, wasn't he? By the time Joe had graduated from college and taken the MCAT with disappointing results, he was convinced there was something really wrong with him. An awful lot of his fellow students seemed to have glided along the path that Joe had carved out for himself, yet he was stalled. It was looking like he might never get into medical school. So Joe decided to have himself evaluated for ADHD. The more he read about it, the more he thought this explained his whole problem. The evaluator disagreed. So did the one from whom Joe sought a second opinion. And the third.

Carrie fell into a similar trap. Identified as "gifted" when young, she had been brought up to believe that she should be gifted in doing just about everything in life. When Carrie started hopping from one type of job to another after college, she and her family decided she might have ADHD, which was the only explanation they could come up with for why she kept failing at jobs that should, according to her IQ, be a snap for her. As it turned out, ADHD wasn't the problem, but anxiety was. Carrie didn't like to admit that she found herself almost paralyzed by fear when she started a new job and that this made it really hard for her to concentrate on her work. Fortunately, the evaluator from whom she sought a diagnosis of ADHD discovered the real problem and was able to refer her to a therapist who specialized in anxiety disorders. This therapist not only offered treatment and coping strategies but helped Carrie accept her diagnosis without shame.

Cal didn't have any particular reason—such as an IQ score or comparison to a peer group—for believing that he had ADHD other than that he was currently in a dead-end job, changed jobs often and impulsively, and had very few friends and no girlfriend. He believed his life should be different and had apparently cast around over the years for an explanation for why it wasn't. My colleagues and I have seen numerous people like Cal, who simply feel that if they're not getting what they want out of life, there must be some psychological deficit at work. None of us can explain this phenomenon; it's almost the opposite of the TV singing-contest shows where the contestant clearly can't stay on key and yet believes rigidly that she's destined for vocal stardom: in this case the person believes he cannot perform well in life when in fact he does perform as well as most people, even if it is not up to his own internal standard.

To adopt a standard for defining the term *impairment* other than comparison with the true norm is like something out of *Alice in Wonderland,* where nothing is as it seems, and words can have whatever meaning one wishes to give them. Saying that a person functioning as well as or even better than the average or typical population can still be considered impaired makes a mockery of the term *disorder* and does a disservice to those struggling with really not being able to function as well as the norm.

If the professional says you do not have ADHD, any of the following could be responsible for ADHD-like symptoms:

- Being over age 55 or perimenopausal, when increased forgetfulness, distractibility, and disorganization are normal

- Recent medical problems, such as thyroid dysfunction, otitis media, sleep disorder or apnea, or strep throat (though this particular connection is rare)

- Excessive recreational drug use (marijuana, alcohol, cocaine, methamphetamine, and so on), which can result in attention, memory, and organizational problems

- Unusual stress, though the ADHD-like symptoms would then be *temporary*

- Injury to the regions of the brain responsible for sustained attention, behavioral inhibition, working memory, and emotional self-control

Any of these possible causes should have been uncovered by the evaluation, and the practitioner should refer you to the appropriate professionals to follow up on them.

Step Two

Change Your Mindset

Know and Own Your ADHD

Having a diagnosis of ADHD is like holding a passport to a better life. It gives you access to:

- **Medication** that will help you concentrate, persevere, manage your time, and resist distractions that pull you away from what you want and need to do—and in doing so significantly reduce your risks for various adverse consequences and thus improve your quality of life and even life expectancy

- **Specific types of psychological therapies** that can target your ADHD-related difficulties and, in combination with medication, optimize management of this disorder

- **Coaching** by counselors and other professionals specializing in life-coaching for adults with ADHD to help them set and fulfill their goals, improve their health and lifestyle, and further maximize the effects of the other treatments

- **Strategies** for playing up your strengths

- **Tools** that can help you compensate for weaknesses

- **Coping skills** that will boost your success in specific arenas, from work to home

- **Support** from peers and experts who want you to realize your dreams and reach your goals

- **Accommodations** in college, other educational settings, or even in your workplace that you may require and be entitled to under the Americans with Disabilities Act

The rest of this book lays out your options for getting each type of help—where to go, what to do, how to use available resources. But that's just half of what you need to make treatment and support work best *for you*. The other half comprises knowing yourself and the ADHD that *you* have. And to know your ADHD, you have to truly own it.

Accepting ADHD as part of your psychological makeup is what I mean by "owning your ADHD." If you merely acknowledge the disorder at some distant intellectual level, paying public lip service to the diagnosis but privately rejecting it, you'll be stuck where you are. People I've seen react that way don't embrace treatment. They've wasted time and money on the diagnosis and end up with the same struggles they've always had.

> **Mental avoidance of the diagnosis wastes enormous amounts of time and emotional energy as well as opportunities for a far better life.**

I find, in fact, that accepting the diagnosis can be rather liberating for adults. They no longer have to play mind games with themselves or others in which they deny, excuse, defend, distort, massage, or in other ways avoid accepting the disorder. I am bald, color blind to reds and greens by about 60% or more, not well coordinated, cannot draw or paint a lick, am not very mechanically inclined or talented, am musically rather inept, now have to wear glasses, have nearly completely gray hair (what is left of it), find the remainder now migrating south into my nose and ears, and am developing a slow but progressive left facial weakness when talking, among other psychological and physical inadequacies I certainly possess. And I am fine with owning them, warts and all. None prevents me from working, socializing, and otherwise engaging my life fully. Because when I decided to own my inadequacies, my next thought was "So what? No one is perfect; big deal. Now just own it and get on with life."

I hope you can do the same: get on with all the learning, loving, living, and leaving a legacy that a happy and productive life ought to entail. Happiness or at least contentment can come only from accepting yourself as you are, and that includes ADHD. Owning your ADHD doesn't have to demoralize you, because when you really own it, you too can then conclude "So what?!" Admit that you have it, accept the diagnosis, own it as you own other features of your self-image, and then you can really begin to work with and master it. You can't work with something you won't own and don't even know much about. So embrace understanding your ADHD, owning it as part of who you really are, and then working to diminish its adverse effects on your life to improve your chances of leading a meaningful, effective, and successful life.

If you haven't accepted that you have ADHD, you can't get all those things listed at the beginning of Step Two that *should* be the benefits of getting a diagnosis. Accepting your ADHD can lead to:

- Being able to seek help
- Discussing ADHD rationally with others
- Evaluating what types of accommodations, if any, you may need at work, school, or home
- Adapting to the condition
- Coping with it as necessary

In my years of counseling adults with ADHD, I've come to believe that reframing your view of yourself and your life to put ADHD in the picture is in fact among the most crucial changes you can make to master ADHD. It's the only way I know to keep ADHD from running, or ruining, your life. Unfortunately, accepting ADHD as part of who you are may be a tall order if you've been trying to explain your problems in some other way or people have been telling you forever that there's nothing wrong with you that couldn't be fixed with a little willpower. Fortunately, changing your perspective on ADHD is not a single leap you need to make. It's a *process*: You start by coming to *know it*, then you *own it*, and finally you're able to *work with it*.

6

Know Your ADHD

Let's start with knowledge about ADHD:

Knowledge Is Power

Read this book. Try to commit to taking the time. I've broken the book down into manageable chunks with lots of visually stimulating callouts, but you can always skip over the boxes, lists, and charts and go back to them later. Set a goal of reading a chapter or number of chapters of text every day—even skimming at first—to be sure you finish it. If you have one, try setting your computer, phone, or wristwatch alarm to remind you to read for 15 minutes at a certain time every day.

Take advantage of the extra sources of information listed throughout this book. You'll also find a comprehensive list in the Resources at the back of the book.

Be skeptical. If you read enough, you'll be able to decide for yourself what makes sense in what you read. To paraphrase another author, truth is an assembled thing, so read widely and rely on a variety of sources, and the most consistent and reliable information will filter through to you. The information at the end of Chapter 11 will help you become better informed without wasting time sifting through misinformation, exaggerated claims, and outright falsehoods.

What Goes Wrong Psychologically When You Have ADHD?

What *causes* ADHD, as far as we know, is neurological (in the brain) and hereditary (in the genes). As the box on pages 103–105 describes, brain-imaging technology is already showing differences in brain development in those with ADHD. We also know that ADHD can arise from brain injuries and not just brain development problems. And we also know from genetic studies—such as studies of biological family members and even identical versus nonidentical twins—that the disorder is highly heritable.

> Brain-imaging technology is a group of methods by which the live brain is scanned to produce pictures of its structures and the activity going on inside.

Studies have shown that you probably inherited ADHD:

- Ten to 35% of the immediate family members of children with ADHD also have the disorder.

- When a parent has ADHD, up to 40–57% of his or her biological children will also have ADHD. This means if you have a parent with ADHD, you are eight times more likely to end up with ADHD than if your parent does not have ADHD. Likewise, if you have ADHD, your offspring are up to eight times more likely to have it also.

Now you can forget about what caused you to have ADHD. It's too late to change that. Knowing what goes wrong as a result of those causes, however, can help you target treatments and coping methods very specifically.

Research that my colleagues and I did over a couple of decades showed us that ADHD causes a lot more problems than can be summed up by the 18 symptoms found in the DSM. Those 18 are used by most clinicians to diagnose ADHD, and yet *we found 91 more* (listed in the Appendix) *that cropped up in a lot of people with ADHD.* That certainly helped to explain why ADHD can be so hard to diagnose. But what did this abundance of symptoms mean? Now that we had identified them, how could we use this long list to understand ADHD better?

My work and that of others has shown that all these problems seem to cluster together into three categories. ADHD appears to be a combination of:

✓ Poor inhibition

✓ Poor self-regulation

✓ Problems with executive functions—those mental abilities that allow us to regulate our own behavior

As you'll discover in the rest of Step Two, these three are interrelated. Poor inhibition leads to poor self-regulation, and problems with executive functions can produce seven different types of self-control problems. *I now believe that it all comes down to self-regulation.* However, I think you'll find it easier to understand your own unique version of ADHD if you look at it within the framework of these three problem areas.

Here's a sampling of the symptoms that fall into these categories. How many do you experience?

Poor inhibition

✓ Find it difficult to tolerate waiting; impatient

✓ Make decisions impulsively

✓ Make off-the-cuff comments to others

✓ Have difficulty stopping my activities or behavior when I should do so

Poor self-regulation

✓ Can't seem to wait for a payoff or to put off doing things that are rewarding now so as to work for a later goal

✓ Likely to do things without considering the consequences of doing them

✓ Likely to skip out on work early if it's boring or to do something more fun

✓ Start a project or task without reading or listening to the directions carefully

Problems with executive functions

✓ Poor sense of time

✓ Forget to do things I am supposed to do

✓ Unable to comprehend what I read as well as I should be able to; have to reread material to get its meaning

✓ Get frustrated or emotionally upset easily

✓ Am poorly organized—my life and things seem in constant disarray

✓ Have trouble planning for and meeting goals I set for myself or carrying out tasks I agree to do for others

This is just a sampling, but I think you can probably see from these examples that **poor inhibition** basically means you have difficulty stopping yourself long enough to think about what you're about to do. Without that pause, you can't exercise much self-control. **Self-control** means any response or set of responses that you direct at yourself and your own likely behavior that would lead you to do something different from what your first impulse would dictate. Think of inhibition as your psychological braking system. You put on that brake and slow down long enough to decide whether the intersection you're approaching is clear and it's safe to drive through, as well as just how effective what you are planning to do is likely to be. Self-control might mean coming to a full stop and waiting till the traffic clears even though you're in a hurry and would like to try to drive unsafely around it.

Executive functions are the specific self-directed actions that we use to control ourselves. They are the mental abilities that we all use to consider our past and then anticipate the future and guide our behavior toward it. They work like a GPS in your brain, giving you the step-by-step instructions that you need to get to your destination. Scientists divide them up and label them differently, but executive functions generally include abilities like inhibition, self-awareness, working memory, emotional self-regulation, self-motivation, planning, and problem solving when obstacles to our goals are encountered along the way. After inhibiting the impulse to act, we turn on these abilities during that pause. It's important to know that using these abilities takes will and effort. They are not easy and automatic. These executive functions help us decide exactly what to do when we exert self-control. Think of them as your mental GPS (planning and self-monitoring your progress) when combined with your gas pedal (motivation), brake (self-restraint or inhibition), and steering wheel (mental guidance).

The Five Areas of Difficulty in Managing Daily Activities

It's easier to see how thoroughly poor inhibition, poor self-control, and executive function problems can invade your life if you look at the difficulties that they cause in the following five major areas. Quickly check off which of these problems you've experienced to get an idea of all the ways ADHD affects you.

Problem Area 1: Poor Self-Management Relative to Time, Planning, and Goals

- ☐ Procrastinate or put off doing things until the last minute
- ☐ Poor sense of time
- ☐ Waste or mismanage my time
- ☐ Not prepared for work or assigned tasks
- ☐ Fail to meet deadlines for assignments
- ☐ Have trouble planning ahead or preparing for upcoming events
- ☐ Forget to do things I am supposed to do
- ☐ Can't seem to accomplish the goals I set for myself
- ☐ Late for work or scheduled appointments
- ☐ Can't seem to hold in mind things I need to remember to do
- ☐ Have difficulty keeping in mind the purpose or goal of my activities
- ☐ Find it difficult to keep track of several activities at once
- ☐ Can't seem to get things done unless there is an immediate deadline
- ☐ Have difficulty judging how much time it will take to do something or get somewhere
- ☐ Have trouble motivating myself to start work
- ☐ Have difficulty motivating myself to stick with my work and get it done
- ☐ Not motivated to prepare in advance for things I know I am supposed to do
- ☐ Have trouble completing one activity before starting a new one
- ☐ Have trouble doing what I tell myself to do
- ☐ Poor follow-through on promises or commitments I may make to others
- ☐ Lack self-discipline
- ☐ Have difficulty arranging or doing my work by its priority or importance; can't "prioritize" well
- ☐ Find it hard to get started or get going on things I need to get done

If you've struggled with a significant number of these problems, it should be pretty clear to you that ADHD in adults is a problem with the ability to organize behavior over time to prepare for the future.

How many of these problems (you may hear people on your treatment team call these "deficits") do you recognize in yourself? Do any examples from your own life come to mind?

_____

_____

_____

_____

Problem Area 2: Poor Self-Organization, Problem Solving, and Working Memory

- ☐ Cannot focus my attention on tasks or work as well as others

- ☐ Have difficulties with mental arithmetic

- ☐ Can't seem to remember what I previously heard or read about

- ☐ Trouble organizing my thoughts or thinking clearly

- ☐ Forget the point I was trying to make when talking to others

- ☐ When shown something complicated to do, cannot keep the information in mind so as to imitate or do it correctly

- ☐ Dislike work or school activities where I must think more than usual

- ☐ Do not seem to anticipate the future as much as or as well as others

- ☐ Have difficulties saying what I want to say

- ☐ Unable to come up with or invent as many solutions to problems as others seem to do

- ☐ Often at a loss for words when I want to explain something to others

- ☐ Have trouble putting my thoughts down in writing as well or as quickly as others

☐ Can't comprehend what I read as well as I should be able to; have to reread material to get its meaning

☐ Feel I am not as creative or inventive as others of my intelligence

☐ In trying to accomplish goals or assignments, find I am not able to think of as many ways of doing things as others

☐ Have trouble learning new or complex activities as well as others

☐ Have difficulty explaining things in their proper order or sequence

☐ Can't seem to get to the point of my explanations as quickly as others

☐ Have trouble doing things in their proper order or sequence

☐ Unable to "think on my feet" or respond as effectively as others to unexpected events

☐ Easily distracted by irrelevant events or thoughts when I must concentrate on something

☐ Slower to react to unexpected events

☐ Can't seem to remember things I have done or places I have been as well as others seem to do

---

Is this list all too familiar? Which problems struck a strong chord with you?

_____

_____

_____

_____

You may know from personal experience that adults with ADHD have significant problems with organizing their thoughts and actions, doing so quickly and effectively, and thinking up multiple possible ways of doing things or overcoming obstacles they encounter in pursuing their goals or assigned tasks in daily life.

Problem Area 3: Poor Self-Restraint (Inhibition)

☐ Find it difficult to tolerate waiting; impatient

☐ Make decisions impulsively

☐ Unable to inhibit my reactions or responses to events or others

☐ Have difficulty stopping my activities or behavior when I should do so

☐ Have difficulty changing my behavior when I am given feedback about my mistakes

☐ Make impulsive comments to others

☐ Likely to do things without considering the consequences

☐ Change my plans at the last minute on a whim or sudden impulse

☐ Fail to consider past relevant events or past personal experiences before responding to situations

☐ Do not think about the future as much as others my age seem to do

☐ Not aware of things I say or do

☐ Have difficulty being objective about things that affect me

☐ Find it hard to see a problem or situation from someone else's perspective

☐ Quick to get angry or become upset

☐ Don't seem to worry about future events as much as others

☐ Don't think about or talk things over with myself before doing something

☐ Have difficulty using sound judgment in problem situations or when under stress

☐ Trouble following the rules in a situation

☐ Not very flexible in my behavior or approach to a situation; overly rigid in how I like things done

☐ More likely to engage in risk-taking behavior than others

☐ More likely to drive a motor vehicle much faster than others (excessive speeding)

Which of these problems are ones you struggle with? Can you think of a time when you've had to deal with these recently?

_____

_____

_____

_____

Notice that these problems with inhibition apply not just to behavior but also to thinking and emotions. This is why poor inhibition and limited self-regulation cut such a broad swath through your life: If you can't stop your own actions, thoughts, and emotions to give time and self-control a chance to get any traction, you won't be guided to decisions that would be better for your long-term welfare.

Problem Area 4: Poor Self-Motivation

- ☐ Likely to take shortcuts in my work and not do all that I am supposed to do

- ☐ Likely to skip out on work early if it's boring or hard to do

- ☐ Can't seem to defer gratification or to put off doing things that are rewarding now so as to work for a later goal

- ☐ Give poor attention to details in my work

- ☐ Do not put as much effort into my work as I should or as others are able to do

- ☐ Told by others that I am lazy or unmotivated

- ☐ Have to depend on others to help me get my work done

- ☐ Do not seem to get things done unless they have an immediate payoff for me

- ☐ Have difficulty resisting the urge to do something fun or more interesting when I am supposed to be working

- ☐ Inconsistent in the quality or quantity of my work performance

- ☐ Unable to work as well as others without supervision or frequent instruction

☐ Do not have the willpower or determination that others seem to have

☐ Things must have an immediate payoff for me or I do not seem to get them done

---

Which items on this list are familiar to you? In what types of situations?

_____

_____

_____

_____

I suspect you know how tough it can be to persist when what you have to do is boring, takes a lot of effort, or is prolonged. If you can't motivate yourself, how can you persist? ADHD leaves you depending on immediate rewards or threats of consequences imposed by others.

Problem Area 5: Poor Emotional Self-Regulation

☐ Quick to get angry or become upset

☐ Overreact emotionally

☐ Easily excitable

☐ Unable to inhibit expression of strong negative or positive emotions

☐ Have trouble calming myself down once I am emotionally upset

☐ Cannot seem to regain emotional control and become more reasonable once I am emotional

☐ Cannot seem to distract myself from whatever is upsetting me to help calm myself down; can't refocus to get into a more positive frame of mind.

☐ Unable to manage my emotions to accomplish my goals successfully or get along well with others

☐ Remain emotional or upset longer than others

☐ Find it difficult to walk away from emotionally upsetting encounters with others or leave situations in which I have become very emotional

☐ Cannot rechannel or redirect my emotions into more positive outlets when upset

---

Which of the preceding problems affect you? How, in particular?

_____

_____

_____

_____

Adults with ADHD find it very hard to inhibit strong emotional reactions and then down-regulate them so they are more acceptable to others and more supportive of longer-term goals and welfare.

My recent studies have shown that 89–98% of adults with ADHD report having major problems in the five problem areas listed on the previous pages, compared to just 7–11% of typical adults in the general population:

	Adults with ADHD (%)	Adults in the general community (%)
Self-reports		
Time management problems	98	8
Poor mental organization	89	11
Inhibition problems	94	7
Self-motivation problems	95	9
Emotional control problems	98	7

	Adults with ADHD (%)	Adults in the general community (%)
Reports of others who know the adult well		
Time management problems	96	9
Poor mental organization	84	7
Inhibition problems	94	11
Self-motivation problems	84	9
Emotional control problems	99	14

These five problem areas created by ADHD in major adult life activities obviously pervade nearly everything you have to do on a daily basis. That they can severely interfere with your education and your functioning in your work ought to be very clear. But it's probably glaringly obvious to you how they have been interfering as well with your social relationships, including dating, marriage, or living with a partner. If you've been having problems with managing money, driving, or raising your children, you may now see how those abilities can be disrupted by ADHD. No doubt you can even see how these problems might deter you from taking preventive health measures and adopting a lifestyle that promotes your overall long-term welfare. These connections point to an inescapable conclusion:

ADHD in Adults Is Not Merely a Trivial Disorder of Attention!

Instead it's a problem with the ability to organize behavior over time to prepare for the future. The five problem areas in ADHD add up to an exceptional disorder of self-regulation that results in a veritable nearsightedness about the future. And that, as you probably know firsthand, is a recipe for disaster in most major life activities.

• • • • •

ADHD is a form of *time blindness*.

• • • • •

What you will learn in the next three steps that can help you tremendously is this:

The problems that ADHD creates are not so much with knowledge, or the back part of our brain, but with performance, or the front part of our brain. That is where we use that knowledge in daily life for greater effectiveness. Thus, the problems for you have more to do with not using what you know at critical points of performance in your life than with not knowing what to do.

Hold on to that thought. It's important not just to your understanding of ADHD but to your confidence that you can improve your life—that you are not stupid, lazy, or "just not paying attention." You know what to do. Let's see how you can learn to use what you know when you need it.

The Brain as a Knowledge versus Performance Device

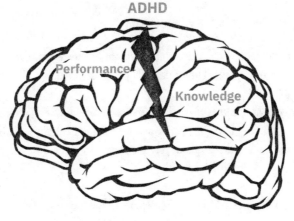

7

Resisting Impulses
The First Step in Self-Control

"Why am I so easily distracted when I'm trying hard to concentrate?"

"I know I was supposed to get that project done this morning, but I just couldn't seem to tear myself away from this great video soccer game I was playing with guys all over the United States. Now I am really in hot water at work. If I find something exciting, fun, or just plain interesting, I get completely stuck."

"I can't tell you how many times I have shot my mouth off without thinking and wound up offending someone, or purchased things I thought I really wanted even though I didn't have the funds to pay them off on my credit card, or just up and quit a job because I was bored with what I was asked to do that day."

We all need to stop and think before we act. And *stop* is the key word here. Thinking before we act so we can choose a wise course of action starts with the ability to wait. If we immediately responded to everything that happened around us, we'd spend our days like human pinballs. *Not* responding to events that happen around us is critical to getting tasks done. That's because most of the things around us are irrelevant to the goals we are pursuing at the moment. Inhibition is the foundation of tact. It helps create a pause in our automatic actions so we can think about the situation and thus make good decisions—and become better and better decision makers over time.

Dragged Away by Distractions

Here's a short list of activities that 30-year-old Dan said he found difficult if not impossible:

✓ Reading

✓ Doing paperwork

✓ Attending a college lecture

✓ Watching TV

✓ Watching a movie

✓ Having long conversations

Dan found reading more than a paragraph at a time almost impossible because there was "always something going on around me that distracted me, whether it was a bird chirping outside the window, one of my kids walking through the room, or some tangent that my mind went off on when I read a sentence that reminded me of something else." Doing paperwork was even more painful: "I can't seem to concentrate on such boring stuff for very long." Lectures? They were "the worst, because I couldn't leave the class when I got bored, but I couldn't keep my attention on what the teacher was saying for very long either." Dan could watch a TV show that he really liked but still found himself "channel surfing across a lot of different programs, especially during the commercials." Dan's wife liked to sit and talk about her day after work, but Dan said he always had to be doing something physical, moving all the time or just being busy. She, of course, took that as a sign that he wasn't paying attention to her needs and so didn't care about her. "Inside," he explained, "I feel so restless even if I'm not actually moving much. I just have this urge to be busy, or touching stuff, or playing with anything around me. It drives my wife nuts."

Do you identify with Dan's list? What would you add to it?

_____

_____

_____

_____

For most of his life Dan has been told he doesn't "pay attention." That never made much sense to him. He doesn't purposely drift off or just space out. Key to understanding ADHD is that many problems labeled simply as "difficulty paying attention" are actually problems with impulse control. It's not just that Dan and other adults with ADHD cannot sustain attention. It's also that they can't resist the impulse to pay attention to something else that enters their field of vision . . . or hearing . . . or thinking . . . *whenever* it enters that field if it is more interesting than what they should be concentrating on at the time. *The problem isn't not knowing what to do (pay attention), but not doing what you know at the right time*—which is to STOP before going off on a tangent or reacting to those distracting but irrelevant events.

Poor inhibition is a problem that develops very early in life in most cases and remains a problem for adults with ADHD across their entire life. Parents, friends, and coworkers have probably been baffled by your inability to block out distracting sights, sounds, and movements for as long as you can remember. They can zero in on the task at hand; why can't you? Do you perceive peripheral noises and sights better than other people? Are you more sensitive to everything that's going on around you? No. People without ADHD can stop themselves from responding to distractions; they do it so automatically that they're not even aware of having made an effort to do so. You, on the other hand, lack that "brake" switch that could keep your mind trained on the task that's most important to you: the one you need to get done right now.

Dan's wife might be more forgiving of his hyperactivity if she knew that the problem arises from poorly timed brain development in those with ADHD. The primary motor system of the brain—the part that gives rise to various and small motor movements—appears to mature too early in people with ADHD. This leads to an excess of motor movements or restlessness. And the higher-level brain center nearby, which governs that motor system and organizes our behavior toward future goals, develops too late, as shown in the National Institute of Mental Health (NIMH) study described on page 111. This means that kids with ADHD have the neurological impulse to move around constantly without the brakes that tell them not to. As development proceeds, the fabulous learning machine called the human brain catches up a bit, and that's why Dan doesn't tumble around his living room as an adult. But it never catches up to the capacity of those without ADHD, and that's why Dan still feels that restless urge to move or to do something all the time.

Dan's problems also have a lot to do with sitting still. Impulse control is highly related to the hyperactivity that is more common in kids than in adults.

More on brain development and self-control in Chapter 9.

Notice that Dan says he feels restless inside all the time. He may now be able to resist the impulse to do somersaults in the living room while his wife is talking—an impulse he couldn't resist at age 10—but he does end up tapping his foot, fidgeting with the kitchen utensils or knickknacks next to him, or feeling so uncomfortably antsy that just trying to focus on his wife's voice makes him scowl with irritation. You can imagine how she interprets this reaction from her husband.

Too Quick on the Trigger

Now look at 25-year-old Shayla's list of "impossible" tasks:

✓ Waiting in line

✓ Staying silent when someone "can't seem to get a move on"

✓ Waiting behind many cars to make a right turn at a stoplight

✓ Stopping herself once she's started talking

Saying she "just can't seem to wait for things," Shayla has missed movies she wants to see because she can't stand in a long line. If several cars are in front of her at a red light when she wants to make a right turn, she just drives over onto the shoulder or the sidewalk right up to the light and makes her turn without waiting. When stuck in traffic, she usually rides the horn a lot to try to get people moving "even though I know it won't usually work."

Where Dan notices what he doesn't get done due to distractions, Shayla's problems with inhibition are more about what she *does* do because she can't put on the mental brakes. Her driver's license has already been suspended once due to her risky driving habits. She has walked out on job after job, sometimes on the very first day, because she couldn't stand the boring parts of the work or anything that involved waiting. In school she was constantly being sent to the principal's office for being a "motor mouth," and as an adult she's often labeled a "boor" or an "egomaniac" because she can't seem to resist monopolizing any conversation. As a teen she couldn't stand waiting till she'd saved enough money to buy the little sports car she wanted. So one day Shayla "borrowed" one belonging to a friend of her father's. Fortunately, he refused to press charges when he reported it stolen and the police stopped Shayla speeding along the highway in it. But things don't always end that well these days.

She has ended up in shouting matches with strangers and alienated friends because she blurts out whatever comes to mind. People describe her as hotheaded, tactless, and just plain "clueless" or "stupid." The truth is that emotional and intellectual problems also come into play in Shayla's unfortunate behavior choices (see Chapter 9), but the trouble starts when Shayla doesn't adequately contemplate or deliberate about her possible actions and their future consequences, valuing more the near-term excitement and smaller, more immediate rewards over the less exciting and more punitive future consequences likely to occur with that choice.

Do you identify with Shayla's list? What would you add to it?

One-Track Mind

The same underlying problem that makes it hard for you to sit still and concentrate or to think before acting can, believe it or not, also make it difficult to *stop* what you're doing. All through school, people thought Jess just couldn't learn. He seemed to make the same mistakes over and over. He would stick doggedly with an effort that everyone around him could see was fruitless. Once he broke off a key in the door of his girlfriend's garage because when it didn't unlock the door he just kept twisting it until it broke. As an adult, he bent a corkscrew beyond recognition because he didn't notice as he tried to open a wine bottle that the metal wasn't a foil covering on top of a cork but a metal cap in the cork's place. His neighbor once called the fire department when Jess let his backyard grill set a shrub on fire because he was so immersed in mapping out a vegetable garden that he got distracted while grilling.

When most people make a mistake in the middle of a project—an ingredient added to a dish doesn't have the effect the recipe said it would, or the paint is almost gone with only half the garage done—they tend to slow down and think for a moment about the mistake and whether it means anything important. Mistakes often give us information about how we could be doing something better or whether we should stop doing this activity altogether, at least for that moment. Adults with ADHD do not seem to monitor their performance of tasks as well as others, or to use mistakes they make to give them important information that could guide their actions in the immediate future. It's as if they start on a straight line and stay on it relentlessly no matter the mistakes that may be piling up behind them.

If what they are doing is particularly fun, rewarding, or interesting, many adults with ADHD may also find it hard to stop even when they're not making mistakes but need to get on with another task that needs to be done soon but is far less interesting. While some advocates for adults with ADHD call this "hyper-focusing," researchers call this problem perseveration. Perseveration often looks like procrastination. But as you might know, it's not that the person has decided to put off something that isn't fun. It's that he or she decided to keep going on something that *is* fun.

Do you identify with Jess's experience? Can you think of similar problems you've had?

_____

_____

_____

_____

• • • • • • • •

The "time blindness" of ADHD starts with a lack of impulse control.

• • • • • • • •

Poor inhibition can make doing any task feel like taking one step forward and two steps back, over and over. It can also make a poor impression on those whom you want to think favorably about you. Knowing this deficit is behind problems you may be having that are like those of Dan, Shayla, and Jess can help you stop beating yourself up. This knowledge can also lead you straight to ways to compensate that can make a world of difference.

Improving impulse control starts with changing your brain: See Step Three.

Compensating is all about buying yourself time: See Step Four.

8

Self-Control

How to Get What You Want

"I have no self-discipline! I have goals, but I never get them done. When things get even the least bit difficult or I run into a problem, I just give up."

"My life is nearly half over, and I haven't been able to accomplish most of the goals I've set for myself. I'm as bright as most of the people I know. Sometimes I wonder if I'm just lazy or don't care as much as others about getting important things done."

"One time a friend and I were working this construction job, and he said he was going to quit that day and drive from Wisconsin to Denver and just look for a new job out there. He had never been there but had heard it was a cool place to live. So I said I'd go with him, just like that. No plans, no job prospects, no place to live— nothing! And we both walked out and started driving. I mean, how stupid is that?"

Lacking self-control robs you of free will. This is one of the most tragic consequences of ADHD. You might think you're doing what you desire. Yet if you can't inhibit your behavior, you miss out on the delay between an event and your response. That delay is essential: It gives you the chance to think. Even more critically, that delay empowers you to *choose freely* among all of your available options, both now and in the future. Len, the guy who spontaneously took off for Denver with a friend, might have felt pretty good—free and easy—when they set out. But it didn't take long for him to realize that ending up in an unfamiliar city with no friends, no job, and no money was *not* what he wanted. Had he taken a moment or two to think it over before acting, he probably wouldn't have gone.

That's what I mean by self-control: the ability to choose something other than your initial impulse so you can get something in the future that you want more or that is better for your long-term welfare and happiness.

Self-control is defined in psychology as any response, or chain of responses, that we direct at ourselves that leads us to change our own behavior instead of just acting on impulse so that we can change what will happen in the future. It is action directed at the self to change that likely future.

This capacity not to respond to events is much more highly developed in humans than in any other species. A deer that smells smoke in the woods will probably run away from the smell without thinking. A person who smells smoke in the woods might pause to figure out whether it seems likely to be a forest fire, a campfire, or a lantern and then act accordingly. "Free will" is just another way of saying we have the capacity to deliberate on our options to act, which in turn gives us the opportunity to choose what's best for us down the road.

With self-control, we can direct our behavior toward the future in general, and what may lie ahead for us specifically, rather than always engaging in knee-jerk actions that might get us nowhere (or might get us to Denver, where we have no future). We can get ready for the tomorrows, the next weeks, the next months, and even the next years in life. We can organize ourselves with an eye on that future.

And in that future, there are many prizes to be had. There are also all those hazards that can be avoided when we can anticipate them and plan well for them. Without self-control, we wind up in places we didn't really want to be, feeling stupid, guilty, or demoralized, lazy or apathetic, not to mention rudderless—and may even end up injured or dead due to reckless risk taking.

> Step Four contains a series of "rules" that you can apply to trick your brain into exerting self-control where it doesn't normally.

The Six Key Processes Involved in Self-Control

You may view *self-control* as a pretty loaded term. How many times since you were a child have you heard the command "Control yourself!"? How many times did you think to yourself that you would if you only had some idea *how*? Understanding how self-control works will defuse the term. You'll also see that self-control is a process with little entry points where using a strategy or tool can free your will so you can get what you want out of life—not just this minute but in the future stretching out before you.

These are the six key components involved in self-control:

1. Self-control is a **self-directed** action. This means instead of acting in direct response *toward* an event, you stop and take action toward yourself. *When his friend said he was going to Denver, if Len did not have ADHD, he probably would have inhibited the "Wow, that sounds great to me too!" response long enough to think about what uprooting himself might actually mean over the longer term. Maybe he would then have made a list of the issues that needed to be considered in such a relocation (such as a job, housing, transportation). Engaging in self-restraint (pausing) is a self-directed action, and so is writing yourself notes to contemplate and break down complex decisions and things to be done.*

2. These self-directed actions are designed to **change your subsequent behavior.** There are seven such self-directed actions (which are our executive functions) that I will discuss later. *Len might have decided to nod and say, "Good luck!" Or he might have chosen to say, "Wow, that sounds great to me too, but maybe I could come out after you tell me whether it's panning out for you." Or maybe he would have opted not to take any action right now but have recognized a need to think about it, make some notes to pursue more information on the important issues (job, housing, transportation), and then consider taking action in the future: If moving sounded good but going to Denver right now wouldn't work for a variety of reasons, perhaps Len should start thinking about where else he might want to relocate in the future. Notice that the initial pause and even making a "do list" of issues are self-directed actions that lead to a change in what Len is likely to do next.*

3. This change in subsequent behavior is designed to **achieve a net gain (maximization) of positive outcomes across both the short *and* long term for the individual.** The behavior is directed at the future but will also take the immediate consequences into account to come up with the best bottom line. *Len might have to give up the positive consequence of going on an exciting road trip to get a greater positive outcome later, such as moving to Denver, but only after he had found a job out there. All of Len's self-directed actions lead to a greater likelihood that the decision to relocate or not will be more in line with his longer-term welfare.* With self-control, we sacrifice the bird in the hand for the more profitable two in the bush. Unless, of course, we have adult ADHD, in which case we will keep opting for the bird in the hand and never work our way toward a flock.

> • • • • • • • •
> If it didn't result in a net positive, why would anyone exercise self-control?
> • • • • • • • •

4. Self-control depends on **a preference for larger delayed rewards over smaller, immediate ones.** If you can't conceive of the future or you don't value later consequences, there's no point to self-control and you won't use it. *If Len didn't have ADHD, he might not have to think for more than a second about what he'd rather do—run off to Denver today or plan for a move someplace new over the*

Psychologists have found that our preference for larger, delayed consequences increases from childhood all the way up to our early 30s, paralleling the development of the frontal lobes of the brain—the seat of our self-control. But ADHD derails that development and leaves even adults picking the smaller immediate outcomes, instead of the larger delayed ones.

next year. He'd immediately know that realizing the dream of having a good job and an affordable home in a beautiful new location was more valuable to him than the fleeting fun of taking off on a road trip with a friend without a plan, just to get there right away.

5. Self-control bridges the time lapse between an event, our response, and an outcome. We may not need self-control at all when the gap between event, response, and outcome is small or nil. Imagine your 5-year-old daughter spotting the ice cream truck coming toward her. She asks you for an ice cream, the truck stops, you buy one and hand it to her. She's completely calm through the short sequence of events. Now imagine that your daughter hears the ice cream truck but can't see it. She has to contain her excitement while she figures out whether the truck is coming toward her and how far away it is. By the time it comes into her field of vision she covets that ice cream as if she hasn't had one for years. She jumps up and down and squeals with excitement as she pleads, "Daddy, Daddy, there it is—can I have an ice cream?" Whereupon you say, "Well, an ice cream will spoil your dinner. How about if we buy one and put it in the freezer for later?" It now takes every ounce of self-control a 5-year-old can muster to inhibit the impulse to kick you in the shins. For a 5-year-old in this situation, self-control may involve mainly controlling emotions. For an adult trying to keep working toward saving for a house when there are dozens of opportunities every day to spend that money right then and there instead, all kinds of abilities are required to exert self-control.

> The abilities we need to exert self-control are called *executive functions,* and they're discussed in Chapter 9.

> "Carpe diem"—seize the day—could be the motto of all adults with ADHD. It's great on vacation; it's terrible as a daily rule.

When the time between event, response, and outcome is long, self-control helps us manage ourselves relative to time and the future. It helps us bind these events disconnected in time into a cohesive idea that we can take with us to keep our eye on the prize.

Researchers refer to bridging the gap between event, response, and outcome over long time spans as a capacity for the *cross-temporal organization of behavioral contingencies.* It is job one of your executive brain (frontal lobes). That's a mouthful. Think of it as the ability to engage in time management or, more aptly, to manage yourself relative to the passage of time.

As an adult with ADHD, Len will have a hard time working toward that relocation goal. With the outcome so far off, he's likely to forget about the whole plan and do little or nothing to prepare. He might set a date for moving but be just as unprepared for it when the time comes as he was when taking off on a whim with his friend. Self-control in this case would mean he'd have to push himself to research regions of the United States, spend time every week on job searches in the chosen area, find out how much income he'd need to afford the kind of home he wants, and more—all before reaping the benefits of the move.

Hindsight and foresight rely on nonverbal working memory, a mental faculty in short supply in adults with ADHD, as discussed in Chapter 9.

6. For self-control to occur, we need **the capacity for both hindsight and foresight.** How do we bind the events, responses, and outcomes of life together when there are large gaps in time between them? We have to have a fundamental sense of time—that there is a past, a present, and a future—and be able to conjecture about the future. To speculate about the future, we have to be able to recall our past and evaluate it to detect possible patterns. This recall of the past, or *hindsight,* gives us the ability to think about possible futures that are based on those past events, or *foresight.* It would prevent Len from taking off for another locale without preparation, as he had when he left for Denver.

What you might have thought of as self-control as a child—sitting still when told to, being quiet in class when you really wanted to tell your friend something, eating only one doughnut instead of the whole box—has far greater ramifications in adult life. Paradoxically, without self-control you can't be free. Let's take a look at the abilities that make up self-control next.

Poor inhibition leads to poor self-control and robs you of your free will—the capacity to choose wisely among possible options for responding to events or to your own thoughts.

9

Executive Functions

The Seven Abilities That Make Up
Self-Control . . . and More

"Why does it take me 2 hours to write a business letter that other people can write in 10 minutes? I can't seem to get my ideas to flow in this nice orderly sequence to write down what I want to say."

"I have a terrible time controlling my emotions, especially if something happens that frustrates or upsets me. One of the many times I locked my keys in my car and really had to get somewhere important for my job, I got so angry at myself that I started to tear the door off the car. People driving by must have been staring at me and thinking 'That guy is really crazy!' but I didn't care."

✓ Chapter 7 showed that we use inhibition to delay the decision to respond to an event—to wait.

✓ Chapter 8 showed that this delay gives us time to engage in self-control. Self-control, or better yet, self-regulation, allows us to monitor our own actions, stop ourselves as needed, contemplate our possible actions, and then choose the wisest course of action to get the best possible outcome in the future.

✓ But *how* do we control ourselves? What allows us to use the time created by resisting an impulse wisely? That's the subject of Chapter 9.

Scientists in the field of neuropsychology call the capacities behind self-control the *executive functions*, or sometimes executive abilities. They're the actions directed at ourselves, the mental activities we engage in when we think about our future and what we should be doing to get there and to make it better.

Different scientists have conceptualized executive functions differently, but what you'll read here is the view I've developed. (It is, after all, my book.)

Research now suggests that there are at least six other executive functions *besides inhibition*—a total of seven different actions we use to monitor our own behavior, stop ourselves, think things over, and guide our eventual behavior while controlling our emotions and motivations to optimize our success at attaining our goals. We use these actions for the single purpose of controlling our own behavior to achieve a better future:

✓ Self-awareness

✓ Inhibition

✓ Nonverbal working memory

✓ Verbal working memory

✓ Emotion regulation

✓ Self-motivation

✓ Planning/problem solving

> • • • • • • • • • • • • • • •
> **Knowing which of your executive functions is the weakest will help you understand which type of self-control to target in efforts to cope and compensate.**
> • • • • • • • • • • • • • •

Here's how they develop:

✓ *Executive functions are more obvious in children and more internalized in adults.* We're hardly aware of these mental machinations. No one can really see us engaging in them. They're the things we adults "do in our heads" all day long as we choose what to do in every situation. They are what most of us refer to simply as "thinking." Yet I believe all seven are entirely obvious, public behavior early in child development. Executive functions were likely also public or obvious early in human evolution, when the human brain was much more primitive, but that's a story for my other book on executive functions. As we mature, we internalize them, like the species probably did as it evolved.

Think of it this way: People develop an ability to engage in some action to themselves, like talking out loud to themselves to control their actions. Eventually, these are no longer observable and occur just in the brain, like having an idea. We say these actions are now "internalized," as we are able to inhibit those signals from leaving the brain, entering the spinal cord, and activating the actual behavior. You can now imagine doing something without then actually doing it physically. We come to "privatize" this process, probably through a simple switch deep in the brain that can prevent a thought from being activated via the spinal cord as a behavior. This internalizing or privatizing process creates a private form of action that we usually call "thinking."

Notice that this process involves inhibition; the thought can go on, but the action it might create is prevented from occurring. Now you know why people with ADHD often act out their thoughts impulsively instead of keeping them in their mind (brain) for further evaluation before finally implementing them. If you are into high-tech gadgetry, you know about simulators. They let us do things in a virtual world without really doing them in the real world. Well, that's what this process of privatizing our actions lets us do—we get to simulate our ideas and plans before we actually implement them to see how they might play out and get to learn from such mental simulations. If we couldn't do that, we would likely experience more mistakes, failures, and injuries, and a greater likelihood of death, all of which are real risks for people with ADHD.

These familiar examples will illustrate what I mean:

- Six-year-old Lena puts her hand over her mouth when she wants to tell a secret that her friends just told her not to. At age 16, she won't need the physical restraint; she'll just visualize doing so in her mind and maybe use internal self-talk to stop herself even if she really wants to tell.

- Eight-year-old Rico softly but audibly repeats to himself, "Stay inside the lines" and "Don't push too hard on the pencil" during classroom writing assignments to keep himself focused on the teacher's rules and reminders. When he's older, he'll be able to use his "mind's voice" to say such things to himself so automatically that he may not even be aware that he's issuing his own silent reminders.

- Crissy and her classmates start out using their fingers, some beads, and then a number line on their desk to carry out the steps to solve a math problem. As they mature, they'll be able to complete problems using mental rather than manual manipulation. They can visualize manipulating the beads or moving their hand along a number line without really doing that in the real world.

Adults with ADHD report that they need to use tactics that fall in between obvious, public self-reminders and the nearly automatic mental reminders that other adults give themselves. One adult said he locks his mouth with an invisible key to get himself to stop talking. Do you use tricks like that to control your behavior?

_____

_____

_____

_____

✓ Executive functions operate together but can cause impairments *separately*. Other scientists and I have divided executive functioning into seven separate abilities to understand them better. But we humans don't experience them as separate, nor do we use them one at a time as adults. The executive functions operate like the sections of a symphony orchestra, playing simultaneously to produce seamlessly beautiful music. It is the action of these executive functions *in concert* that permits normal human self-control. When ADHD enters the picture, so do deficits in executive functions. These deficits might occur more in one executive function than in the others, producing different types of behavior problems with self-control in different adults with ADHD. This means *there are really seven executive functions or seven different types of self-control and so seven different kinds of deficits in ADHD*. Knowing which one is the biggest problem for you makes it easier to choose external tools and strategies that can make up for those internal deficits. Later in the chapter, you'll have a chance to review the problems listed under each executive function to get an idea of where your biggest problems lie.

✓ *The seven executive functions develop one at a time, in sequence, each added to the earlier ones to build a mental structure, like a Swiss Army knife, that gives us a set of mind tools that facilitate our self-control.* As each executive function develops in a child, control over the child's behavior gradually shifts in four important ways that should ultimately add up to adult self-determination:

- *From external to internal:* We all start out as babies being controlled by purely external events—a loud noise, a mother's departure, a wet diaper, or, much later, the commands and directives of our parents—and then we become increasingly managed by internal forms of information, much of which deals with the past and future (images, self-speech, motivation, and so forth, which make up our hindsight and foresight).

- *From others to the self:* At first, we need to be controlled and managed entirely by others (such as parents), gradually becoming able to better control ourselves.

- *From the present to the future:* When very young, the only thing that matters to us is what's happening right now. Throughout childhood we become increasingly aware of and directed toward future events. Think of how long you'd expect a typical 3-year-old to think ahead and plan out her day compared to how far in advance a 14-year-old should be able to do it (a day or two) and then for what period a 36-year-old should be able to do so (6–12 weeks ahead).

- *From instant gratification to deferred gratification:* More and more as we mature, we find the big prize at the end of the long haul to be worth waiting and working for and so turn away from the small seductions and rewards of the moment to work for those much bigger rewards.

Think of what people usually mean when they call adults "childish." The barbs usually start flying at adults who seem ruled by whatever is going on around them, who need other adults to do their thinking for them, who don't think ahead, and who have no patience.

Sound at all familiar? Does an example from your own life come to mind?

_____

_____

_____

_____

As an adult with ADHD, you've been subjected to delayed development of each of the seven executive functions. You're no child, but these lags make you less effective than other adults and may make your peers treat you as if you were a child. You can head off blame (including self-blame) and help yourself make these shifts from child to adult functioning more fully if you know a little more about how the condition disables each executive function.

Self-Awareness—Using the Mind's Mirror

Even though I focused so heavily on inhibition above because it is so essential to self-control, it is actually not the first executive function to develop. Self-awareness is the first executive function to emerge in childhood. It goes hand in glove with inhibition because neither one makes any sense without the other right alongside it, which means they both likely develop together or at least very close in time. The other five executive functions would be useless without these first two: If you are unaware of how you are behaving, why would you and how could you stop yourself from behaving the way you're behaving? And if you don't monitor your behavior and change it as necessary, you're also not likely to spend time thinking about your past and future, how they can inform your decisions going forward, and even what goals you want to achieve.

That is actually what the vast majority of other species of animals do on this planet. They are stimulus-response creatures, reacting to the moment as events overtake them and adjusting their behavior only after the fact as a result of the consequences—if they survive them. But not us. For we humans know that simply reacting is not what is best for us if we want to optimize our *long-term* welfare, quality of life, and even survival over our short-term actions and their immediate rewards.

First We Need to Be Aware of Our Surroundings

After we are born, our first order of business in development is to start to attend to our surroundings and then begin to orient our motor responses to the things that we detect are happening to us. We then start to adjust our next response based on the actual consequences of what we do. All animal species do this, because if they don't, they won't survive for very long as adults.

Then We Need to Be Aware of Ourselves

But very soon after developing such outer-directed attention and behavior, human children turn that process of attention to themselves. After all, they and their behavior are also part of the world they inhabit, and so it makes sense that they should begin to become self-aware. As this ability emerges, we, unlike the vast majority of other creatures, can see our reflection in a mirror and recognize ourselves. This mirror test is precisely what is used by scientists to determine if a species is self-aware and also when in human infancy this awareness starts to develop.

One likely reason we develop self-awareness and other creatures don't is that we are one of a rare handful of species that survive by living in groups with others, some of whom are kin *but others of whom are not!* You probably don't realize just how very special living in that niche is. Most other social creatures don't live with beings they are not genetically related to, but we, chimps, dolphins, and a very few other animals do. To do so requires some sort of frontal-lobe executive system for tracking them and monitoring how we reciprocate with them as well as how they reciprocate with us. Working memory, to be discussed later, is well suited for doing just this.

In the niche of rare social species that live with non-kin, it becomes important to monitor what you do, how others react to it, and whether they repay the favor. We then adjust our behavior accordingly so that we can alter what we do before we do it. We routinely depend on others, including non-kin within our tribe, for our survival. But we don't naively trust everyone, because non-kin do not always have our best interests at heart the way biological family members usually do. Thus how we control ourselves—to improve our social interactions, networks, and welfare, sharing with the trustworthy reciprocators while quickly detecting and avoiding the cheaters and exploiters—gives us a competitive advantage over others (and other species) that are not doing so.

What Does This Mean for People with ADHD?

Regardless of its initial evolutionary function, self-awareness is so crucial to human survival and social success that we frequently take it for granted. But when a disorder like ADHD undermines this basic executive function of self-awareness, it can undermine the entire system of self-regulation and its purpose. A deficit in that executive function means you have less awareness of how you're acting, how your behavior is coming across to others around you, and what the predictable consequences would be for acting that way. You have more difficulty directing your attention to yourself than others do. This may lead you to barge into social situations or be offensive without realizing it, and not to notice how others around you are reacting. Both adults and children with ADHD are often less aware than others of how loudly they're talking, how much they're talking, what they're trying to say, how much they're moving while saying it, why they're even saying it (rambling and forgetting their goals), and especially how others are reacting to what they're saying. Three of the ADHD symptoms in the DSM-5 diagnostic criteria in the Appendix (and the only ones representing impulsiveness) illustrate precisely this problem of verbal heedlessness.

Now extend this poor self-monitoring to other types of behavior and especially social interactions besides verbal ones and you can see the myriad social problems this limited self-awareness can create for you. Compound this deficit further by the fact that you might not realize how emotional you're becoming during some social exchanges, and you can see how your social life can go off the rails very quickly. Unfortunately, those with whom you're interacting don't necessarily know you have ADHD—or understand its role in causing your behavior—and may see you as immature, self-centered, or egotistical. They don't understand that you can't stop yourself if you can't monitor what you're doing and how it is playing out with others.

This poses a sizable problem for both loved ones who can see what you cannot see—that your behavior may at times be inappropriate and that others are judging you negatively for it—and professionals who deal with adults with ADHD: How can they help someone who doesn't know he has a problem or doesn't think it's significant enough to be addressed? It is for this very reason that a new requirement was added to the DSM-5 diagnostic criteria: Now clinicians must corroborate the reports of what the patient is saying with others who know the patient well or, if not available, with archival school and other records that may reflect how impaired the patient's functioning is. Until age 30 or older, even adults with

ADHD cannot be trusted to be the sole judge of their own behavior, symptoms, or impairments; they simply do not have the necessary self-awareness to make accurate self-assessments. You may feel belittled by a helping professional who gathers information from others on your behavior rather than trusting your own reports. Try to understand that the professional is following guidelines that will help diagnose your problems and lead to treatment. The deficit in self-awareness can obviously cause you a lot of problems. It may delay your recognition or acceptance of the fact that you have a disorder—and in turn delay your seeking or receiving the help you need and deserve. It doesn't have to be that way.

Nonverbal Working Memory: Using the Mind's Eye

Nonverbal working memory is the third executive function to develop, just shortly after your ability to monitor your own actions and then to inhibit the immediate urges to act. It's the capacity to hold information in mind—not through words but through your senses. So this executive function allows you to hold in your head pictures, sounds, tastes, touches, and scents. Because vision is our most important sense for survival, nonverbal working memory largely represents the ability to engage in visual imagery—to "see to yourself" in your mind's eye. A close second in importance is hearing, so we can also "hear to ourselves" using nonverbal working memory. More accurately, we resee past events and rehear past sounds and the things others have said to us. But we can also resense all of our other senses if we need to, such as smell (when I recall the aroma of a good wine or scent of a favorite flower), or taste (as when I recall or retaste my favorite lamb or salmon dish), or even refeel the soft texture of my favorite flannel shirt on my neck and arms. It's all resensing in our mind as we recall these past sensations. So while I focus here on visualizing and rehearing things in our mind, don't forget we can do that with our other senses too.

How Nonverbal Working Memory Guides Us

1. We get a map that leads us to the future we want. Seeing to ourselves means reseeing past relevant events. What we've seen sometime in the past we can see again in our head, thanks to this executive function. What we've heard before we can hear again, also in our head. Resensing past experience, which constitutes our "ideas," creates an internal stream of information through our mind that we can use to guide our behavior across time toward a goal. By envisioning our past, we can foresee a possible future. It works just like the GPS in your car. The device brings up a map of your region and allows you to use it to get to a particular destination, which is your goal. Images of past relevant events are the maps that we can use to guide us to our goal.

2. We gain the powerful tool called *imitation*. When you can hold an image in your mind of what you have seen and experienced, especially if it involved watching another person do something novel, you also now have the power to imitate the behavior of others. Instead of having to go through the hard knocks of trial-and-error learning in every new situation to come up with that new way of doing something, you can call up your mental picture of how Dad or your best friend handled a particular problem beautifully. And then you just copy that image of what they did. No trial and error, no failure and frustration, and no harm to ourselves. Imitation gives us a cheap and easy way to acquire new behavior without learning it directly. We just "photocopy" what we saw someone else do. How cool is that? It's important to understand that when you learn through non-verbal working memory, you don't necessarily copy the other person's actions literally but rather copy your image of those actions. The image is a template you can use to copy what they did. Yet you always put your own spin on what you learn from others. Nonverbal working memory also enables you to do the opposite of what others have done rather than imitate them in everything they do, when what you saw them do failed or resulted in errors, punishment, or harm. You just do the opposite or do nothing at all and thus avoid whatever harms befell them. Imitation, or more accurately vicarious learning, lets us take the best of what other people have learned to do while avoiding the worst of their own mistakes, thus making for a very efficient form of social learning that humans have elevated to an art form during their evolution. Now imagine how inefficient and even harmful learning will be if you don't use nonverbal working memory very well if at all. We see such problems in people with ADHD, who seem to benefit less than most people from what they see others doing around them.

> Nonverbal working memory allows not only imitation but the opposite: staying away from what someone else did that proved ineffective. This is called *vicarious learning*.

3. We can foresee the consequences of our actions. Chapter 8 explained that self-control depends on both hindsight and foresight: We need to be able to see in our mind's eye both our past experiences and any pattern that sheds

Hindsight → Foresight → Preparation to act

light on our likely future experiences. Hindsight brings your pertinent past history forward into the moment to inform you of the best way to behave given what happened to you before. Foresight, or forethought, means taking any patterns perceived in images from the past to anticipate what will happen in the future.

4. We gain self-awareness. We use our visual imagery to study our past, or even just to hold our immediate past behavior in mind, so we can monitor our own actions. Then we can compare them against what our plans, goals, and strategies were and evaluate how well we are doing in performing that task or achieving our goals. We gain a greater self-awareness of our life across time.

5. We're capable of sensing the flow of time and thus managing ourselves relative to it. The ability to hold a sequence of past events in our mind and refer to them across time appears to give us a *sense of time* itself, how it is flowing or progressing, and how best to manage our behavior relative to it. We understand how much time may have passed, how much we have left, and what we need to do when necessary to get tasks done on time. We can judge how long something might take, such as driving to work on a rainy morning, and thus plan our departure so as to get to work on time. This capacity to sense and judge the flow of time and manage ourselves relative to it, which we call *time management,* is one of the strongest predictors of educational and occupational success.

> • • • • • • • • • • •
> **Nonverbal working memory gives us a sense of time, a key to time management.**
> • • • • • • • • • • •

6. We learn to defer gratification. To value a delayed consequence, you must have a sense of the future and use it to guide your behavior. The more you use that sense, the more likely you are to focus on the big rewards down the road rather than the immediate, smaller prizes.

7. We can see further and further ahead. As hindsight and forethought develop, we gain an expanding window on time (past, present, future) in our conscious mind. It even gives us our subjective sense of time and its passing. Small children can't see much past a few minutes ahead. And they can't judge time intervals very well, much less use them to coordinate their actions. But by adulthood (ages 20–30), behavior is typically organized to deal with events 8–12 weeks ahead, and our sense of the flow of time is almost continuously informing our decisions and actions. And this time horizon can be extended further into the future if the consequences associated with those events are particularly crucial to us.

8. We value cooperation and sharing. The golden rule may not seem like an obvious product of nonverbal working memory or visualizing to yourself. But when you think about it, it makes perfect sense. With a grasp of the past, you remember what others have done for you and you for them, and with your sense of the future you realize that sharing and social cooperation insure you against possible shortfalls of resources. Therefore you're willing to give up and share some excess resources now with a less fortunate friend or family member in the hope that the recipient will share abundance with you later, when you may need it. This voluntary and reciprocal form of altruism is what makes social groups so effective in surviving and competing against less cooperative individuals or groups. Selective and voluntary sharing with like-minded people in our social group is like an insurance policy against future misfortunes in life.

> **Nonverbal working memory may be what makes selfish altruism part of human nature.**

How ADHD Interferes with Nonverbal Working Memory

To get an idea of which type of self-control you might target when selecting strategies from Steps Four and Five, think about which of the following are the biggest problems for you.

✓ *You have little or no feel for the passage of time, have trouble judging how much time activities will take, and cannot manage yourself well relative to the passage of time.* When nonverbal working memory and its related sense of time are disturbed by ADHD, it can leave an adult without a typical sense of time. All that seems to matter to you is what is happening now. So you live much of your life in the now rather than getting ready for what is going to happen next. It can also leave you with a sense that time is passing much more slowly than it really is. This can make you feel like you have a lot more time to get things done than you actually have. It may cause you to waste time doing things that are irrelevant to your goals or tasks. Events, deadlines, or the future itself generally arrive much sooner than expected and catch you off guard, often leaving you in a panic or a crisis.

✓ *You can't reactivate a large number or wide variety of past events.* Typically, the more children mature, the greater the number and variety of past events they can conjure up. But the lags caused by ADHD keep the capacity for visual imagery and rehearsed experiences fairly primitive. This deficit in nonverbal working memory creates a major gap in the resources that adults with ADHD have to guide their behavior compared to typical adults. So to others you might look like you don't think before you act. It would be more accurate to say you have trouble *remembering*—or more accurately, *resensing*—before you act.

> *Sam is known to friends as tactless because he blurts out whatever comes to mind; he can't read social cues because he doesn't attend to them and thus has no archive*

of such images to serve as a repertoire of subtle facial expressions and what they communicate.

✔ *Long, complicated sequences of behavior may pose a serious challenge for you.* Knowing how to behave in delicate social situations, sticking with the rules of a complex game, completing a multistep task like filing a tax return—all of these typical adult scenarios may leave you with no clue because your brain has difficulty holding all those mental images.

Sebastian's hyperactivity as a child kept him out of the team sports he loved, so he thought he'd join the company softball team to make up for lost time. He no longer got tagged out for constantly leading off a base, but from inning to inning he'd forget how the opposing players hit, who was a fast runner, what the status of the game was, and how his own team members fielded. So he was always in the wrong place at the wrong time and led his team in errors. After being benched for a couple games he quit the team.

✔ *Vicarious learning may not be so available to you.* If you have trouble learning from the successes and mistakes you've observed in others, you're stuck learning everything the slow, painful way: by yourself, on your own, through trial and error.

Claire's coworkers sometimes wondered whether she was taking drugs. Otherwise, how could she have failed to notice the reaction others got when they interrupted the boss at a meeting, took too long to return a customer's call, or missed a report deadline? When she complained bitterly about being barked at in front of everyone for these transgressions, they all wrote her off as "either an idiot or stoned."

✔ *You have little foresight.* If you can't hold past images in mind long enough—or hold enough of them—to see patterns developing, you won't be able to predict what's likely to happen next and get ready for it.

Mike had gotten enough tickets to have the image of a flashing red light approaching his car from behind emblazoned on his brain. Yet when he impulsively drove 30 miles per hour over the speed limit to get to his night class on time, he couldn't predict that he'd get stopped again—but he did.

✔ *Self-awareness comes slowly to you.* If you can't monitor how you're doing, whether in a routine task or a social situation, it's not easy to see where you are in relation to your long-term goals. You may not get the mental signals that it's time to chart a new course when that old one is not taking you where you want to go.

Sonya really wanted a lasting relationship. But whenever she was at a party, she'd drink too much, get too personal with strangers, talk incessantly so that no one got a word in edgewise, and make cracks about other women's outfits. Any guy she met who was interested at first drifted off quickly. When Sonya got home at the end of the evening, she invariably looked at herself in the mirror, pronounced herself "hot," and then brooded about why all the guys were such "losers."

✓ *Without a strong sense of the future, you'll opt for the quick reward, sacrificing gradual accumulation of assets.* You'll be like the grasshopper who whiles away the summer singing while the ant stores food for the winter, or the first little pig who quickly built a house of mere straw while his more self-controlled sibling took longer but built his house more substantially of brick. When the winter arrives or the wolf is at the door, the quick shortcut is never as good as the effort to pay attention to the longer term.

Tim and Marie were on the verge of divorce. Tim claimed he wanted to buy a house as much as his wife did, but every time they went on vacation, he'd listen to some time-share pitch and end up signing a contract for a week at yet another resort that Marie didn't necessarily want to return to. At the rate they were going, the couple wouldn't be able to buy a house until they were 70, unable to save for a down payment after these "investments."

✓ *You may not make a good team player . . . or know how to be a good friend.* When the grasshopper was starving, the ant rebuked him for failing to think ahead and create a nutritional stockpile. Social insurance can save your life. But if you have no concept of the future, sharing what you have with others makes no sense. All you can appreciate at the moment is the loss of your own hard-earned assets. You can see where this is going for adults with ADHD: You may have little capacity for or interest in sharing, cooperation, turn taking, and repaying the favors of others or fulfilling the promises you've made to them. They may very well respond to your requests for help as the ant did to the grasshopper.

LaTonya didn't understand why so many of her friends didn't return her phone calls. Her friends complained to each other that she was awfully quick to bum a ride or ask for another favor or even money but never hesitated to say no when one of them needed help from her. She owed every one of them a small amount of money but consistently claimed she couldn't afford it when a friend was short of cash and asked if LaTonya could pick up the tab for a fast-food burger. Many of them eventually became ex-friends.

> **Which of the preceding difficulties are big ones for you?**
>
> _____
>
> _____
>
> _____
>
> _____

Verbal Working Memory: Using the Mind's Voice

The next or fourth executive function to develop in children that facilitates self-control is the ability to talk to yourself, especially in your mind. As kids we do this publicly. We narrate our play, talk to ourselves when alone, and weigh our decisions out loud. As every parent knows, kids can be pretty free with their commentary, even though their remarks may not be too flattering. Gradually children begin to talk to themselves silently, though they may still move their lips. By ages 7–9 they suppress even those movements, and now this voice occurs entirely in their mind. From this point on, the voice in our head will accompany us through all our waking hours until we die.

How Verbal Working Memory Guides Us

I also refer to this as the mind's voice. The capacity to converse with yourself, especially mentally, in concert with the capacity to sense to yourself brings about another form of self-regulation and with it a number of important features for self-control:

  1. It allows us to describe and contemplate an event or situation. Let's say you come home from work and say hello to your roommate, and he doesn't answer. Nonverbal working memory might tell you that the look on his face indicates he's not happy. With verbal working memory, you might put words to the way he could be feeling: "He's angry." But that's still a global and vague sense of the situation. You might then use your mind's voice to look for more information by asking yourself specific questions, such as "Is he angry at me, at his girlfriend, his boss, or someone else?" Describing the situation to yourself and even interrogating yourself with such questions gets you much more specific information than just a mental image might achieve and could head you away from a hasty "What's wrong with you?" and toward a more nuanced and socially sensitive reply. You might say to yourself, "He's not glaring at me. He's just stomping around the room looking mad. Last time it turned out he was just ticked off that he had missed a short putt while golfing that morning or had to work that weekend."

2. It makes problem solving possible. With private speech we can interrogate ourselves about our past to figure out how to solve a current dilemma. In trying to figure out how best to respond to your aggravated roommate, you might ask yourself, "What happened last time I assumed he was mad at me?" This introspection might reveal that you picked a fight, which your roommate was all too happy to engage in so he could take out his ire on someone. Your conclusion might then be that you need to find a way to ask him what's wrong without being either defensive or offensive.

3. We can formulate rules and plans. We need verbal working memory (our mind's voice) to examine how things went in the past and extract from that rules for making sure they go well in the future. Our self-questioning and other self-talk allow us to weigh pros and cons based on our past experience, to talk to ourselves about what we could change to improve the future, and to set out steps toward a goal. Our rules might involve diet and other lifestyle matters, social conduct, spending or saving habits, and more. Often, we make our self-statements and rules external and easier to follow by writing them down on a to-do list to help us remember and use later.

Eventually we go further and generate a hierarchy of rules about rules (called *meta-rules*). An example of a meta-rule in government might be the procedure required for enacting new legislation. In a school, it might be that the criteria for expelling a student must be approved by the school board. An example from daily life is the six well-known steps to solving a problem: (a) state the problem specifically, (b) list as many solutions as you can, (c) critique each one for its utility, (d) select the one most likely to achieve your goal, (e) implement it, and (f) evaluate its success. They are simply rules used to discover other, more specific rules that apply in a specific situation.

4. We can follow rules we're given. Using nonverbal and verbal working memory together, we call up mental pictures of similar situations from the past and then ask ourselves whether a rule we've learned applies here. If we don't really want to follow the rule anyway, we might use self-talk to either persuade ourselves to obey or convince ourselves that this is one of those exceptions that make the rule. Our self-speech complements our visual imagery by allowing us to get much more information out of our thinking than an image alone can convey.

5. We can hold in mind what we have silently read to ourselves or heard others say. In school it was called *reading and listening comprehension*. In the adult world it's necessary in most of what we do. We need to understand and remember what we've read in reports and heard others summarize at work. We need to grasp the rules and procedures at our kids' school so that we don't put the kids at a disadvantage. If a bill goes unpaid, we need to comprehend the consequences explained in the statement and what action we must take to avoid the financial and legal fallout.

6. We're capable of moral reasoning. The rules—laws, ethics, customs—of the culture we live in play an important role in guiding our behavior. If we don't know what they are and can't talk to ourselves to remember what they are and how to apply them when we most need them, we can end up on the fringes of society, if not ousted altogether.

How ADHD Interferes with Verbal Working Memory

Is verbal working memory the type of self-control that eludes you most?

✔ *You talk out loud too much, especially when interacting with others, and often get off on irrelevant tangents:* Verbal working memory is based on our capacity to talk to ourselves using our inner or mind's voice. We can simulate what we will say, practice it, and then edit or change it as needed so that when we do say things to others those things are more tactful and hence more likely to promote the relationship and our own welfare. ADHD delays this ability to think and talk to ourselves privately in order to consider what we are about to say to others. So a lot of verbal thinking is done out loud, publicly, and is often inappropriate for that context. This can cause you to ramble on and on while freely associating to whatever thoughts come into your mind, to interrupt, and to verbally intrude on others' interactions. All of these behaviors can be interpreted as rudeness and lack of consideration for the feelings and intentions of others. And because of the reduced capacity for self-awareness and monitoring that is also inherent in adult ADHD, you may not even be aware of how you're coming across.

✔ *You don't use self-talk to control yourself or solve problems.* Without the benefit of self-talk, you shoot from the hip all the time. You might make a lot of false assumptions about people's intentions because you don't examine your first impression. You might literally attack any problem rather than thinking it through.

You might go through roommate after roommate and end up living alone.

✔ *You let events and the environment rule.* If you can't use self-speech to formulate your own rules and plans, you're always at the mercy of the moment. You're also vulnerable to the influence of others, whose advice and directives substitute for your own self-determined rules of behavior.

Hien was a "good kid" according to his teachers and his parents. But as he became independent, he seemed increasingly subject to bad influences. There was always someone at the local tavern who would convince Hien that he could buy another round. There was always a whim that would carry Hien into some ill-advised decision even though later he agreed with his parents that he should have known better.

✓ *You have trouble setting your own standards and making your own plans.* Without visual imagery and the ability to question your own past behavior, you won't extrapolate a list of dos and don'ts for future use.

Nina struggles with her weight, but she can't seem to resist a tempting dessert or snack when she sees it, so she keeps eating a diet that adds pounds to her frame. Without verbal working memory along with nonverbal working memory, Nina can't connect her impulsive eating habits with her weight gain or stick to a diet.

Carmelita is tired of being broke, but when she has paycheck in hand, she can't seem to stop shopping. If she could reflect on the consequences of those actions, she might be able to talk herself into going to the bank first and depositing a portion of her check in her savings account or even having her employer do this automatically.

Both women have occasionally tried to make rules to help themselves. Nina decided to severely limit her consumption of fat and sugar. Carmelita decided to put $100 from each paycheck into her savings account. The problem was that neither of them could make adjustments when their plans didn't work out. Nina's diet made her feel so deprived that she "cheated" constantly and never lost weight. With verbal working memory to aid her, she could have eventually created a meta-rule that before she went on any diet, she would go see her physician and get advice on a sensible weight-loss routine and then remove the most fattening substances from her home so they were simply not available and she wasn't forced to show self-restraint around them. Carmelita found that her savings account was growing way too slowly. With verbal and nonverbal working memory, she could have decided that she would review her spending/saving plan every month to see where she could save more and spend less and also have her employer deposit her paycheck automatically, even setting aside a portion in her retirement plan that the employer would match.

✓ *You follow certain rules rigidly.* A rule is not doing its job unless it can bend a little. The world does not operate on absolutes. But if you can't talk to yourself about the pros and cons and review with yourself the particulars of the situation that you're in, you might follow a rule so rigidly that it will backfire. People with ADHD often lack flexibility.

Max heard that certain fish contain toxic levels of mercury, so he's decided he won't eat any fish no matter what type or what its source. He looks foolish to friends and has offended people who have invited him over or taken him out for dinner, and he gets indignant and nasty when questioned.

Kaye has a set of workplace rules that she follows religiously because she doesn't trust her instincts. For each type of task, she follows the rules that she has developed on her own or been given outright by her supervisors to be sure she doesn't go off course. Following these rules prevents anxiety from consuming her at work . . . as long as the rules never change. It takes her a long time to adjust when new rules enter the mix or replace old ones.

✓ *. . . Or you don't follow them at all.*

Miguel knew that if he got one more speeding ticket, he'd lose his license. The only way he could muffle his instinct to floor it was to try calling up images of his previous tickets, picture what it would be like to be barred from driving, and continuously talk himself into staying below the speed limit. He didn't do that, and now he has to get up 2 hours earlier to take the bus to work.

✓ **You might commit crimes and violate ethical and moral codes.** Many of society's rules and customs are unspoken. Without verbal and nonverbal working memory to help you discern them, you can go through life without a clue, breaking customs and offending your fellow citizens left and right. Laws are written down, but without the mind's voice to remind you of them, you might easily yield to impulse and do whatever you want. And end up behind bars.

Sasha knew it was against the law to steal a car, but that the "joy ride" she and her friends took in the neighbor's unlocked sports car was a felony never entered her mind at the time. All she thought of at the time was that he wouldn't miss it for an hour or two.

✓ **You don't comprehend what you're exposed to as easily as others—whether it's what you read, see, or hear.** The give and take between verbal and nonverbal working memory is what makes it possible for us to make sense of all the input we receive from the world around us. Without that, we miss out on many, many mental connections.

Of course Eric could read. But there were holes in what he took from his reading. His own work was pronounced "sloppy" by his boss because he could quote statistics from various reports but often got things backwards when he drew conclusions from the data. He sent his son to school on a field trip day without the permission slip, the bag lunch, or the swimsuit required; his son had to stay at school with a

younger class. The family's electricity had been turned off twice because Eric for-
got to pay the bill and then didn't notice the deadline for disconnection or the hefty
reconnection fee.

What types of verbal working memory problems interfere with *your* life?

_____

_____

_____

_____

Self-Regulation of Emotion and Self-Motivation: Using the Mind's Heart

The fifth executive function that develops is the self-regulation of emotion. Emotions are primitive yet powerful signals we give off to ourselves and others as to our current feelings, intentions, and state of arousal. But they are also strong motivators of our subsequent actions. They can arouse us to act or prevent us from acting. They can tell us to fight or send us into flight. They can signal within and outside of us our impatience and anger, or joy and affection. If we have no control over our emotions, we have a lot less control over what we do. Emotions arise whether we want them to or not. They are triggered naturally by external events of all kinds. Sadness is triggered by loss (or anticipating loss). Anger is triggered by unfairness, humiliation, unmet expectations, or unanswered needs. Joy is triggered when our expectations and needs are not only met but exceeded and when our desires are fulfilled.

But it's not just external events that bring on emotions. The resensed experiences and self-talk made possible by nonverbal and verbal working memory also have emotional overtones. Picturing your spouse might bring on a feeling of love; talking to yourself about some injustice you recently suffered can make you feel rage.

Fortunately, nonverbal and verbal working memory are also instrumental in helping us regulate our emotional response. We can use self-talk to deliberate with ourselves about how we feel and what we should do about it. We can use our visual imagery and self-speech to try to alter an initial emotional reaction that might cause problems for us, especially if that initial response pushes us into regrettable behavior.

> **Many adults with ADHD say they would be sunk without self-talk. They also find using visual imagery very beneficial but say it requires practice, practice, and more practice. What's been your experience?**
>
> _____
>
> _____
>
> _____
>
> _____

How Self-Regulation of Emotion Guides Us

1. We can control our own arousal. By *arousal* I mean the urge and energy to act, or activation. Emotions are intended to spur us into action. But what if those emotions are exaggerated? Or they are based on a misperception of the situation? In those cases we're obviously going to overreact or go off half-cocked in some way. Controlling our initial emotional reactions to events can prevent us from doing something rash. Or it can drive us to act when we may be suffering from inertia or just plain boredom with what we need to get done. With emotional self-regulation possible, we now have three executive functions that can interact, each supporting the other. Holding on to the images of the past and our visions for the future and being able to talk ourselves down can ensure that emotion doesn't derail our plans and supports our actions toward a better future, even in the absence of immediate rewards. Being able to dampen emotional arousal means we won't start "talking crazy" to ourselves and change course without serious consideration. Being able to visualize our goals and how we will feel when we get there can sustain us through the most boring or unrewarding of immediate activities necessary to get there.

2. We can motivate ourselves when we don't have external rewards to push us. Call it drive, willpower, persistence, determination, stick-to-itiveness—what have you. I call it the mind's fuel tank because it generates the internal "fuel" or drive that powers us toward our goals. While I and many other neuropsychologists think of this as a separate executive function (the sixth here in my list), I combine it with emotional self-control because that is what helps to create our self-motivation. The former is therefore indispensable to the latter. By regulating and even creating our emotions with the other executive functions discussed above, we endow ourselves with internal motivation when no one else is handing us any incentive from the outside. Again, it's the four earlier executive functions working *in concert* that allow us to both self-regulate our emotions and then motivate ourselves to keep going when the going gets tough (or boring). Let's say you want to volunteer with an organization devoted to protecting the environment. You make phone call after phone call asking people to support a major recycling effort. Before long you're extremely dejected at all the rejections you get. In that case you use two of the executive functions you already have (visual imagery, self-talk) to remind you of your successes so far, keep your eye on the ultimate goal, and push you to keep making those calls. If envisioning your success and the potential for reaching the goal isn't enough to get you to pick up that phone again, maybe you intentionally conjure up images of the destruction of the planet and use the anger these images stimulate to motivate you onward.

3. We can make sure we express emotion in socially acceptable ways. This is a biggie. Because we expect adults to have this executive function, society reacts pretty negatively to extreme or exaggerated expressions of emotion. We accept the fact that babies scream at the slightest emotional pain because it's a self-preservation mechanism. And we understand perfectly when 3-year-olds throw a temper tantrum when they don't get the candy at the grocery store checkout counter. But we're embarrassed and disapproving of an adult who bursts into tears or yells in anger in public over a minor frustration like having to stand in a long line at the supermarket.

4. We have a sense of mastery over ourselves and especially our emotional reactions to events. When we develop our capacity to regulate our emotions in the service of our goals and longer-term welfare, we gain a sense of command or mastery of our impulsive reactions to events around us. No longer a slave to our passions, we, and not any potentially provocative events, are in charge of what we will decide to do in response to what is happening to us. We don't go off like a string of firecrackers in reaction to the sequence of events around us because we have self-discipline. We aren't entirely controlled by the flow of events going on around us but instead can exert control over our feelings and reactions as well as over the events themselves. We take charge of our lives instead of life taking charge of us. This makes us less mercurial, unpredictable, or capricious in our responses to events and to others and more measured, stable, and mature, with a new sense of freedom in our interactions.

There's a reason we use the expressions "emotional turmoil" and "emotionally charged" to capture the loss of control one can have when emotionally powerful events trigger strong feelings in us and the internal disarray we can feel when we cannot master those strong reactions to events. Emotion is so powerful that it's as if it has an electric charge that is transferred to those around us. We're expected to keep it under control so as not to impose our feelings on other people. If we are able to regulate our own emotions, when we are angry, we can "go to our happy place" by using images of positive past experiences and talking ourselves into calming down before we finally react to some emotion-laden event. Responding impulsively to our first emotional reactions to events is rarely a good idea if we want to make or keep friends or intimate partners, much less a job.

Do you use images of positive past experiences to "talk yourself down" when angry, anxious, or stressed? Accomplishments that you're proud of—whether it's climbing a mountain, finishing a detail-filled report, or getting along with everyone at a family wedding—leave you feeling both calm and motivated and are great candidates for visual imagery. What are yours?

_____

_____

_____

_____

To put it more plainly, this executive function lets us:

✓ Soothe ourselves when we are having extreme emotional reactions to an event

✓ Use our own mental images and words to distract ourselves from the powerful stimulus that has set off our strong emotional feelings

✓ Consider and implement an alternative emotion by calling up images and words associated with more positive emotions and relaxation

✓ Choose a more moderate emotional tone or reaction that is supportive of rather than detrimental to our own longer-term goals and welfare

This is what emotional self-control is all about: helping us stop and moderate those powerful knee-jerk emotions and substitute others that are more mature, socially acceptable, and consistent with our longer-term welfare.

How ADHD Interferes with Self-Regulation of Emotion

Is it *emotional* self-control that eludes you most?

✔ *Your emotional reactions to events are as impulsive as the rest of your behavior and can make you an outcast.* Without the ability to put on the brakes, you don't have time to alter your initial emotional reactions. Without well-developed verbal and nonverbal working memory, you have less capacity for the visual imagery and self-speech that can help you calm your emotions.

> *The first characteristic Jay's friends use to describe him is "hot-headed." They've all witnessed embarrassing displays of sudden anger from Jay at the slightest provocation, whether it's a pizza delivered with the wrong toppings or a stranger giving him "a look" (that no one else can even see). His emotional hair trigger has cost him social invitations, the trust of coworkers, and a lot of friendships.*

✔ *Emotional reactions that are disproportionate to the event often steer you wrong.* I'm not talking about abnormal, irrational, or grossly inappropriate reactions. But exaggerated emotion that's not in keeping with the situation—laughing loudly at a mild pun made quietly at a funeral, sobbing after a minor snub—can lead to social rejection. Disproportionate emotional reactions can also throw you off course. Feeling extremely angry about a minor failure at work could cause you to leave a job ideally suited to your career goals. Plunging into despair can paralyze you when you really need to keep moving. Becoming elated by modest success can convince you that you've reached your peak, and you might stop trying to achieve a goal that you really value.

> *Vanessa was so ecstatic about her first-ever sales award that she skipped into her boss's office and announced that she was going to start her own sales company and hoped the boss would consider hiring out the company's sales work to her new firm. Her initial excitement is understandable, but her unmoderated display of it to her boss borders on the grandiose.*

✔ *You find it tough to rouse yourself to do what you need to do.* Emotion is definitely a double-edged sword. You want to keep exaggerated and impulsive emotion under control. But you also want to be able to call emotion into play to kick yourself into gear to get things done. You're more subject than other adults to frustration, boredom, and resentment. These tendencies already make it hard to stick with tasks. Add in the difficulties you suffer with attention and concentration and it's even harder to see a task through. Here's where emotion can serve you well. If you can regulate your own emotions, you can use them to kick-start yourself to do work or to maintain your general arousal level so you can stay awake, alert, and focused when you have goals to pursue.

Does emotion run away with you more in some situations than in others? Which ones?

_____

_____

_____

_____

These are the situations where you'll have to resolve to pull out your whole bag of self-talk and visual imagery tricks to stay in control.

Planning and Problem Solving: Using the Mind's Playground

If we can hold images and words in mind, we eventually develop a means to manipulate them. We can take them apart, move them about, and recombine them into new arrangements or sequences in our heads just for the sake of seeing what the results are likely to be. It is our imagination. And it is no surprise that humans do this more than any other species. This is fundamentally a form of mental play, and it originates, I believe, in the extended period of manual, physical play that all children go through as an important stage of early development. Play is simply taking things apart and recombining them just to see what happens or what you wind up with when you do so. It begins with manual manipulation of objects in childhood and progresses to the manipulation of images and even words in your mind. Mind wandering, fantasy, and mental play are the wellspring of human creativity, ingenuity, and problem solving more generally. Where others species can only act and thus suffer from any mistakes they make, humans can mentally simulate a variety of possible options for actions, testing each out in their mind for their likely consequences and ideally choosing the optimal. Where other species may be harmed or even die from their mistakes, we let our simulated ideas die in our place.

Similarly, we play with words as children and then play with combinations of words in our minds as adults. Both of these forms of play, visual–spatial and verbal, lead to novel recombinations of the material we're playing with. Most of those recombinations are junk. (Think of some of the "crazy" ideas we all come up with and then discard when trying to get out of a tough dilemma: "Maybe this cop won't give me a ticket if I tell him I was speeding because my wife is in the hospital about to have a baby" . . . "If I stay up all night tonight *and* tomorrow, that should give me enough hours to write that report that's already overdue" . . . "I could just stand up *both* of the women I made a date with for Saturday, and then neither one of them would think I preferred to go out with someone else!") But some are new ideas or ways to solve problems that lead to new (and even great) inventions or innovations.

> • • • • • • •
> **Play is training for inventiveness in adult problem solving.**
> • • • • • • •

How the Ability to Plan and Problem-Solve Guides Us

1. It helps us consider all the options. Planning entails the ability to generate multiple options for responding to a future event. When we make ourselves aware of all the possible ways to respond, we're much more likely to identify and then pick the best one. Think of brainstorming. This executive function is the best way to prevent the after-the-fact regret of "Why didn't I think of that?"

2. It helps us decide on the best sequence of actions to reach a goal. In the form of mental play that we call planning, we take apart and recombine information in our mind. Once we've got a comprehensive list of options, we can look at the steps each one might involve and then shuffle those steps around to see what sequence will be best. We can, in a real sense, mentally simulate these various sequences to see how they might actually play out before selecting the one that best meets our objectives.

3. The capacity to mentally manipulate information and play with it in our minds gives us an incredible capacity for goal-directed creativity and innovation. Thinking outside the box just can't happen without the mental play that this executive function makes possible. It's like free will (see Chapter 8) cubed. Not only do *you* decide what to do, but you do it in a way that might not have occurred to anyone else. Creativity and innovation may mean a faster route to where we want to go, less effort, or just a better result.

> • • • • • • • • • •
> **Ironically, the planning that you may find painfully slow can help you get a project done far faster.**
> • • • • • • • • • •

How ADHD Interferes with Planning and Problem Solving

Are your problems with self-control connected to an inability to plan and problem-solve?

✓ *You can't think on your feet.* Yes, I know: People usually view your tendency to react fast as a negative. But thinking on your feet means choosing a wise course of action quickly when the need arises suddenly, as it so often does in daily life. Not only is it tough for you to hold lots of information in mind (because of deficits in working memory), but without the planning/problem-solving executive function you can't manipulate the information quickly to plan out possible courses of action or to problem-solve your way around obstacles. This doesn't mean you don't decide quickly—you do! That's the problem—you don't deliberate over all the possible options available before making that snap decision.

> *James desperately wanted to be a firefighter. But when the preliminary training began, it was immediately clear that he couldn't make the quick decisions necessary to save a building or its inhabitants.*

✓ *You can't get or stay organized.* Even when circumstances don't call for a snap decision, you're going to have trouble keeping materials and data organized. This goes for everything from the documentation for your tax return to your files at work or your diabetic child's medical records. If you can't do the mental play, it's hard to envision the game board when you need to make your moves.

> *Every couple of years Marta decided to redo her family's personal financial files because she could "never find anything." She would yank everything out of the file drawers and start trying to come up with her own system. But invariably she quickly got lost in all the paper, and her husband, Guillaume, would come home to find files and documents scattered everywhere.*

✓ *Putting ideas in the correct order is a big challenge for you.* Keep in mind that when you take something apart, you have to put it back together in a certain order for it to operate correctly or make sense. Ideas need to be assembled in their correct order so that they function as intended to solve a problem or make sense. Reasoning, problem solving, planning, explaining, writing, and otherwise conveying your ideas rapidly and in a logical sequence are all going to be tough tasks for you.

> *Writing and giving instructional presentations was almost impossible for Luis. This deficit was really holding him back in his career until his boss realized at one seminar how positively the participants responded to Luis personally. Thanks to an insightful supervisor, the seminar presentations were recast so that a coworker went over the instructional steps and Luis provided the anecdotes and inspirational material. The seminars were more successful than ever.*

Planning and problem-solving skills are central to many adult endeavors. Deficits in these areas can make you feel inadequate if you don't remind yourself that it's not your intelligence level that's the problem; it's the interference of ADHD. What feelings of inadequacy can you now see as the unfortunate fallout of ADHD?

_____

_____

_____

_____

The Seven Executive Functions That Foster Self-Control

The mind's mirror (self-awareness)

The mind's brakes (inhibition)

The mind's eye (nonverbal working memory)

The mind's voice (verbal working memory)

The mind's heart (emotional self-control)

The mind's fuel tank (self-motivation)

The mind's playground (planning and problem-solving)

10

The Nature of ADHD and How You Can Master It

• • • • • • • • • • •
Anyone who tells you all you need to do is buckle down and pay attention should read Step Two of this book.
• • • • • • • • • • •

I hope you can now see that ADHD in adults is not merely a trivial problem with paying attention! Instead it's a far-reaching problem affecting the most important human capacities: It's a condition that robs you of the ability to ignore impulses. It's a deficit in the brain's executive functioning that makes it very difficult to regulate and organize your behavior over time to prepare best for the future.

Nearsighted to the Future

To put it simply, you and other adults with ADHD are blind to time—or at least myopic. You're not lacking knowledge or skill. Your problems lie in the executive mechanisms that take what you already know and the skills you already possess and apply them to more effective behavior toward others and the future. In a sense, your intellect (knowledge) has been disconnected from your daily actions (performance). You may know how to act but may not act that way when placed in social settings where these actions would benefit you.

• • • • • • • • • • • • •
ADHD is a disorder of performance— of doing what you know rather than knowing what to do.
• • • • • • • • • • • • •

Your lack of a sense of time has debilitating, even heartbreaking, effects. You probably don't prepare for predictable events until they are practically upon you—if at all. This pattern is a recipe for a life of chaos and crisis.

• • • • • • • • • • •
You don't *choose* to skip planning or to bypass forethought. Your predicament is not your fault.
• • • • • • • • • • •

96

You're left to squander your energies dealing with the emergencies or urgencies of the immediate moment when a little forethought and planning could have eased the burden and likely averted the crisis.

Dealing with Your ADHD: The Big Picture

This description of ADHD tells us that the strategies and tools that can help you most will be those that help you *do what you know:*

✓ Treatments for ADHD will be most helpful when they assist you in doing what you know at the *point of performance* in the natural environments where you conduct your daily life. That point is the place and time in your life where problems may be occurring because you don't stop and think before you act and thus don't allow what you know to be activated, come forward, and help guide your choices.

✓ The farther away in space and time a treatment is from this point, the less likely it is to help you.

✓ Assistance with the time, timing, and timeliness of behavior is critical. This means modifying your environment to help you do what you need to do when you need to do it. It also means keeping your scaffolding or aids in place.

Fit the Solution to the Specific Problem

Chapters 7–9 described seven types of self-control you might struggle with to different degrees. All of the following guidelines for designing effective treatments, strategies, tools, and coping methods can help you address deficits in the executive functions. In choosing your own aids or accommodations, however, you might pay particular attention to those aimed at the deficits you identified with most.

✓ *Implement ways to become more aware of your actions and to inhibit or adjust them as warranted.* Addressing the deficiencies in self-awareness caused by ADHD is no easy matter. In children, repeatedly reviewing video taken with a smartphone that shows the child's behavior while doing homework, playing with others, or engaging in some other activity has proven helpful to children with ADHD and even autism spectrum disorder. But it's not likely to work for adults. Another thing we do for children might, however, be adaptable. This is transition planning. Before a child engages in a new activity or enters a new social situation, a parent or teacher stops the child, reviews the rules for the upcoming situation with the child, has the child repeat them back, and then reviews what consequences will ensue for obeying or not obeying the rules.

You might be able to recruit a family member or your partner to do something similar, softly inquiring before an upcoming important situation how you would like to act in and get out of this new situation. Your partner could even gently offer some additional tips for achieving those outcomes. You two could also agree to some sort of nonverbal cue or even a single word that only you two know is a signal to stop, become more aware of what you are doing, check out how others have been reacting to you, and adjust your behavior accordingly. For instance, if my voice became too loud at dinner parties (a common problem for me), my wife would give me a subtle signal (lightly putting her index finger to her lips if I was looking at her, gently kicking my shin under the table, or even nudging me with her elbow), which was usually enough for me to quickly soften my voice. You could do the same in many such situations.

Similarly, you could ask a coworker or friendly supervisor if you can meet several times a day to discuss your goals and review your progress toward them. We are more likely to behave better, progress in our work, and even improve in our other self-change programs (exercising, losing weight, quitting smoking, and the like) if we make ourselves accountable to a trusted other for doing so.

✔ *Externalize information that is usually held in the mind.* This simply means putting key pieces of information into some physical form and putting it where the problem now exists so you can see it immediately when in that situation. Stop trying to use mental information so much and back it up with the support of some visual aids or cues.

If your boss or someone else has given you a set of instructions for getting something done over the next few days, stop trying to carry this around in your head and remember it over that period of time. That won't work with ADHD. Instead, always carry a small journal and pen or your cell phone in your pocket and instantly write down the task, any steps given to you to get it done, and the deadline. Then

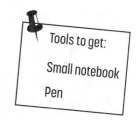

Tools to get:

Small notebook

Pen

keep this in front of you where your work is to be done over the next few days to serve as your external working memory—your reminder to get it done. If you are into technology, think of this as offloading the demands on your mental working memory onto some other storage device—in this case, paper or your cell phone. You can even translate this plan into smaller steps and insert them into your day planner or to-do list as goals for each hour of the day and of the next few before the work is due. The specific technique or external storage device here is not what is important—the principle behind it is!

Tools to use—any of the following:

Kitchen timer

Computer appointment reminders

Smartphone alarms

Day planners/calendars broken down by hours

✓ *Make time physical.* ADHD makes you concentrate mainly on the moment, taking your focus away from the signals and internal sense that time is passing. Use kitchen timers, clocks, computers, calendars, smartphones, tablets, and any other devices that can break time down by the hour and issue alarms when a chunk of time has passed. The more external you make the passage of time and structure that time with periodic physical reminders, the more likely you are to manage your time well.

✓ *Use external incentives.* Arrange for frequent external types of motivation to help get you through any job. For instance, break your project into smaller steps and give yourself a small reward for completing each hour or half hour of sustained work. Motivational "prostheses" are nearly essential to your fulfilling longer-term projects, assignments, personal plans, or social promises. Whether the reward is getting a quick cup of coffee, tea, or a soda to take back to your work area, briefly checking on the status of your favorite sports team on the Internet, listening to a short tune on your

Rewards to consider:

Coffee, tea, soda

Check your favorite team's status on the Internet

Listen to a short tune on your phone or other device

Any small edible treat (as in candy, a cookie)

music player or radio, or even just giving yourself a treat, arrange small rewards for completing smaller work quotas instead of waiting until the work is all done.

✓ Normalize the underlying *neurological deficits in the brain's executive system.* To date, the only treatment that shows any hope of achieving this end is medication. The ADHD medicines (see Step Three), such as stimulants or the nonstimulants atomoxetine or guanfacine, can improve or even normalize the neurological substrates in the executive regions of the brain that likely underlie this disorder and their related networks. The medications do not reverse these deficits permanently; they do, however, have a remarkable positive effect while they remain in your system.

Caution: Going on the Internet to check one thing like a sports score can lead to looking up 67 things. This is why knowing your own ADHD is so important: This reward may not be the right one for you!

✓ Replace distractions with physical cues or reminders to focus on the task at hand. Use whatever physical prompts will keep your mind focused on the task and goals at hand.

There is no scientific evidence for the effectiveness of intervention outside the points of performance in your life where your major problems occur. Avoid talk- or insight-oriented therapy, psychoanalysis, weekly group therapy focusing on complaining, and similar treatments.

Cues to use:

Cards

Lists

Signs

Sticky notes

✓ *Externalize your rules.* Make the rules into physical lists. Post signs, lists, charts, and other aids in the appropriate school, work, or social environment and frequently refer to them while you are in those situations. You can even talk out loud in a low voice to yourself and state these rules aloud before and while you are in these situations. You can also use a device to record and play back these reminders (using earphones to avoid distracting others!).

✓ Break down any task that includes large time gaps *into smaller chunks spaced more closely together.* For instance, rather than accept a project that must be done over the next month as is, break it down into much smaller steps and do a step a day toward that eventual goal. That way, each step does not seem so overwhelming. And you can stay motivated using immediate feedback and incentives for completing each step.

You'll meet all these guidelines again, in the form of rules for everyday success in Step Four and applications to particular areas of your life in Step Five. The more you ingrain them, the more effectively you take charge of adult ADHD.

✓ Stay flexible and be prepared to change your *plan.* As with a chronic medical condition such as diabetes, a treatment plan is made up of lots of interventions that provide symptom relief. But over time, symptom breakthroughs and crises are likely to occur periodically. Don't be afraid to change course—ask for help in doing so whenever you need it—and look for new ways to compensate for the deficits ADHD imposes on you. It's only what you deserve.

Never stop looking for ways to compensate. You never know everything, so try to remind yourself not to get too confident once you start making progress in working with your ADHD.

With these major ideas in mind, you are now ready to master your ADHD. Never forget that with proper assistance—including education, counseling, medication, behavioral strategies, hard work, advocacy, and the support of family and friends—you can make significant and possibly dramatic improvements in your life.

11

Own Your ADHD

Now you know your ADHD. Are you ready to own it?

Being able to identify with the symptoms, impairments, and deficits you've read about so far can make it easier to accept having ADHD. You can even develop a sense of humor about it. But that doesn't mean it won't take time. Many people need to adapt to the idea that they have this condition and that it's not going to go away. Are you having any of these reactions?

✓ Are you in denial about having ADHD? Initial denial is not so unusual but getting stuck there is usually a result of having been coerced to get an evaluation.

✓ Are you feeling a sense of profound relief? Finally knowing what you have and how it accounts for your lifelong struggles can alleviate a lot of self-blame and allow you to stop rehashing the past and get on with the future.

✓ Did you feel demoralized or depressed at first? It's perfectly natural to feel sad about having a chronic, incurable condition. But knowing how much help is available is a great antidote.

✓ Do you feel angry and frustrated? You might feel this way for various reasons, especially if you've gotten inaccurate diagnoses for years. Resentment over all that wasted time and all those unnecessary struggles is natural. The antidote is getting the help you deserve now that you know what's wrong.

✓ Are you sad *and* angry? If ADHD has damaged your life in ways that can't be repaired, you might alternate between these emotions. You may have to work your way through these reactions, possibly with the help of a counselor, to free your energies for improving the future.

It's hard to let go of the pain of lost relationships, jobs, education, and overall well-being that you've suffered as a result of untreated ADHD.

Fortunately, your future does not have to look like your past. If you're feeling strong grief, especially if it seems to be sticking around, some counseling sessions with a professional can help you understand, vent, and resolve these reactions. Then they stand an excellent chance of being replaced by acceptance and hope. Still need some help to own your ADHD? Then take a look at the TED Talk "Failing at Normal" (*www.youtube.com/watch?v=JiwZQNYlGQI*), the YouTube video *Jessica McCabe and Rick Green Get Real about ADHD* (*www.youtube.com/watch?v=wxMpajLtu_g*), where McCabe and Canadian comedian Rick Green take a humorous approach to owning their ADHD while conveying important ideas of how to accept it and cope with it. Or see more videos from Jessica McCabe's YouTube channel, *How to ADHD*.

• • • • •

Your future does not have to look like your past.

• • • • •

An Explanation, Not an Excuse

You are not a victim. ADHD is not an irreparable handicap. The fact that you're reading this book says you are looking for answers, not excuses. But some of the people around you may be inclined to view you as a less capable individual because you have this condition. They may believe it's OK not to hold you accountable for your actions now that you have an official diagnosis. I'm sure you don't want to be treated that way any more than someone in a wheelchair would. Your job going forward is not to excuse yourself from the tasks made difficult by ADHD but to seek out the ADHD equivalent of wheelchair ramps into a building—making accommodations in your physical environment so you are less impaired by your ADHD in various settings. Ramps don't correct a disorder, but they do reduce or eliminate the impairments or negative consequences that can occur from that disorder. Find those ramps whenever you can and build them into your life. The alternative is to wheel around and go back home defeated.

Not only should no one excuse you from the immediate or future consequences of your actions, but you should actually take action to tighten up that accountability by making consequences more frequent, immediate, and salient. You'll succeed best when held accountable for your plans, goals, and actions more often than others are across the day so you receive more frequent feedback.

So, make (and accept) no excuses! Own your ADHD, own its consequences, and then seek to minimize or eliminate those disastrous delays in life that are preventing you from being as effective, productive, and successful as people who don't have ADHD. Find your ramps or build them as necessary, but don't quit on your plans and goals.

Having ADHD Is Not Your Fault . . . but Accepting It Is Your Responsibility

We now know that you probably came by ADHD through a combination of biological and genetic factors, as summarized below. We are also very close to being able to conclude unequivocally that ADHD cannot and does not arise from purely social factors, such as child rearing, family conflict, marital difficulties, insecure infant attachment, television or video games or other "screen time," the pace of modern life, or interactions with peers.

The good news is that this means having ADHD cannot possibly be your fault. The less good news is that it also means there is no cure. You can't get rid of the underlying condition by changing your diet or your surroundings. Nor can you alter any factor in your life in the hope of protecting your children from ending up with ADHD. You can, however, drastically reduce the effects of ADHD on your life. Take Step Three (medication) and you may improve the underlying neurological problems significantly. Then take Step Four and find out what else you can do to change your life for the better.

What the research shows about the causes of ADHD:

- Studies of twins and families have made it abundantly clear that heredity and other genetic factors are the major causes of ADHD. If a child has ADHD, nearly one out of three siblings will also have ADHD. A study done at UCLA examined 256 parents of children with ADHD and found that in 55% of these families, at least one parent was affected by the disorder.

- An estimated 75–80% of variation in the severity of ADHD traits across people is the result of genetic factors, and some studies place this figure at over 90%— higher than the genetic contribution to personality traits, intelligence, and other mental disorders such as anxiety and depression and just slightly less than the genetic contribution to individual differences in height.

- Several recent studies have scanned the entire human genome searching for genes that carry the risk of ADHD. Twelve were found that had a robust or reliable association with risk for ADHD. And other studies indicate there may be at least 10 to 15 or more other sites on chromosomes that are likely to be associated with ADHD. It is therefore likely that ADHD arises from a combination of multiple risk genes, with each contributing a small likelihood of risk for the disorder. The more risk genes you inherit, the greater the number and severity of ADHD symptoms you will have, and the greater the probability you will be impaired by and diagnosed with the disorder.

- A very small number of cases are caused by early-development (often prenatal) neurological injury, such as alcohol exposure during pregnancy, premature delivery (especially with minor brain hemorrhaging), early lead poisoning, stroke, and brain trauma, to name just a few.

- The frontal lobes, basal ganglia, cerebellum, and anterior cingulate cortex are 3–5% smaller, substantially less active, and far more variable in that activity in people with ADHD than in others of the same age.

- Studies show that the brains of those with ADHD react to events more slowly than the brains of those without ADHD. People with ADHD have less blood flow to the right frontal region of the brain than those who don't have ADHD, and the severity of symptoms increases the more blood flow is reduced.

What the research says about popular myths regarding the causes of ADHD:

- Available evidence suggests that sugar plays no role in the disorder and that fewer than 1 in 20 preschool children with ADHD may have their symptoms worsened by additives and preservatives, and even then, only by food coloring, not other types of additives.

- No compelling evidence exists to support the claim that ADHD results from watching too much TV, playing too many video games, or spending too much screen time on your smart devices, though people growing up with ADHD may be more likely to watch television, play video games, or use visual media due to its highly reinforcing quality. Indeed, 15–20% of teens and young adults with ADHD may qualify as having a gaming or Internet addiction.

- Little evidence has emerged that child-rearing practices can cause ADHD. There is no question that families with children who have ADHD show more conflict and stress than other families. But researchers found that this was largely due to the disruptive impact of the child's ADHD on family functioning and also to the likelihood that the parent also had ADHD.

Shaping Your Environment Will Help You Manage Your ADHD

Steps Four and Five are largely about using strategies to help you compensate for the symptoms that medication can't erase entirely. But what they really do is help you tweak your environment to make it workable for you.

As an adult with ADHD, you probably feel like you've been hit with a double whammy: Your symptoms make routine tasks twice as hard (at least) for you as for other adults. And the world doesn't seem too inclined to mold itself around your needs. As I've said before, you can defuse whammy number one to a great extent with medication (Step Three). As to whammy number two, no, the world is generally not going to volunteer to remake itself for your purposes. But there's a lot you can do to control your environments so that they *do* meet your needs:

✓ You can choose to operate in environments where you stand the best chance of success.

> A list of jobs and careers that might capitalize on your strengths can be found in Chapter 25.

  • Can't deal with a pencil-pushing, number-crunching job? Aim for jobs that capitalize on your personality, your physical energy, or your gregarious nature, like sales or the performing arts.

  • Consider becoming an entrepreneur within your company or one who is self-employed. In such creative endeavors, you can indulge your penchant for new or far-fetched ideas. Some of your ideas may lead to novel and profitable innovations for your employer or your own company.

  • Love the world of literature or medicine but can't deal with the detail? Find the department that emphasizes travel and meetings. Adopt workplace strategies that help you get through the grunt work you can't avoid. See if you can hire an administrative assistant who can manage the paperwork and other boring but essential tasks that may be part of your profession. Recruit a mentor among your supervisors who will help you devise less conventional methods for meeting the company's goals.

  These are just a couple of examples of the countless ways you can carve out a friendly daily environment.

✓ You can surround yourself with people who help you play up your strengths and support your efforts to compensate for weaknesses.

  • Your softball teammates may be the most fun people you know, but if you're always the last to leave the postgame beer fests, maybe you can ask a teammate to cue you when you had your one- to two-beer quota.

- If members of your family of origin always expect the worst from you, keep your distance for a while . . . and then go back to the family gatherings once you've got a track record that proves you're the trustworthy adult that Steps Four and Five can help you be.

✓ You can find the best resources available for those with ADHD *and then use them, use them, use them.*

- Throughout this book I'll steer you to time-tested, scientifically proven treatments and sources of professional help. There's more out there for ADHD than almost any other mental health condition that affects adults.

- Feel like someone else is always telling you what's fact and what's not? What's right for you and what's wrong? What you should do and what you should avoid? You can be as well informed as you want to be. On the following pages you'll find tips and resources for sifting through everything you'll read and hear about ADHD to get at the truth. And the truth really can set you free.

A Consumer's Guide to ADHD

I hope that reading about the nature of ADHD in Step Two has made you think not just about your particular symptoms and the impairments they've caused you, but also about who you are aside from ADHD: not just your mix of symptoms and impairments, but your personality, intellectual abilities, physical attributes, talents, living and working environments, and the resources available to you. Then you'll be able to take all the general information on ADHD you are learning throughout this book and conform it like shrink-wrapping to your unique life circumstances.

Take Advantage of the Information Out There . . .

Reading this book is a great start toward educating yourself about ADHD, but it should not be the end. The information available on ADHD in adults could fill many books of this length. So, read widely, listen to experts (and talk to any that you can), ask questions, visit the most informative websites, follow up further on what interests you, and pull together as much information about

Sources of ongoing updates on adult ADHD include:

Resources at the back of this book: Start with a few books, view a few DVDs, then move on as desired to any of the thousands of journal articles in print, which you can find using Google Scholar as a browser to search science journals, or go into the settings of that browser and have it email you weekly with a list of the latest research articles published that week and their links..

Lectures posted on the Internet: Many university psychiatry or clinical psychology departments make some or all of their weekly seminars (called "grand rounds") available on the department's website. YouTube has a number of my lectures on ADHD that were posted by conferences, hospitals, or universities where I delivered them.

Websites of nonprofit organizations dedicated to ADHD: Listed in the Resources at the back of the book.

The professional who diagnosed you: Ask what continuing medical education programs and materials he or she uses to stay current on ADHD in adults and where they can be obtained.

ADHD as you have time to find. Truth is an assembled thing. It comes from no one book, source, expert, guru, DVD, or website. The more widely you pursue information, the more able you will be to distinguish trustworthy information and reliable sources from the fashionable, sensational, flimsy, baseless, or outright false.

. . . But Take It with a Grain of Salt

I probably don't have to tell you to be a skeptic. The controversies that surround ADHD and the claims and criticisms from uninformed sources in the popular media have probably left you ready to doubt what you hear. Great! This tendency will serve you well as you seek knowledge. Question the material you find. Look for or ask for the evidence behind the assertions. Especially challenge claims about treatments that seem too good to be true (they usually are). By seeking the evidence behind the claim—for example, using Google Scholar to browse science journals—you not only evaluate the truth of the

> The more information you seek, the easier it gets to spot the truth.

information you are consuming but also broaden your knowledge base about ADHD and related topics. Sort out for yourself what makes sense, what seems to be the consensus of the clinical and scientific experts who specialize in the disorder, what other adults with ADHD have found to be of value to them, and what fits most appropriately for *your* ADHD.

How do I know when a claim is based on real scientific evidence?

Claims about treatments, causes, and other aspects of ADHD (or any other condition) can sound authentic even when totally unfounded. Here are some clues to whether or not the information is reliable:

Check out the source:

- *Does the source stand to profit?* If the information is tied to a product or service for sale, think of this as more of an advertising pitch than a public service message. Aside from pharmaceutical company ads, this can also apply to any advertising about devices or other methods claiming to drastically improve or cure ADHD, such as neurofeedback, omega-3 or -6 supplements, transcranial magnetic stimulation, and especially cognitive

A few major organizations that are always good sources of information:

Children and Adults with Attention-Deficit/Hyperactivity Disorder (CHADD): *chadd.org*

Attention Deficit Disorder Association (ADDA): *add.org*

ADD Resources: *addresources.org*

ADD WareHouse: *addwarehouse.com*

World Federation of ADHD: *adhd-federation.org*

ADDConsults: *addconsults.com*

Learning Disabilities Association of America (LDA): *ldaamerica.org*

National Attention Deficit Disorder Information and Support Service (ADDISS), Great Britain: *addiss.co.uk*

Canadian ADHD Resource Alliance: *caddra.ca*

Centre for ADHD Awareness, Canada (CADDAC): *caddac.ca*

rehabilitation apps and games that you play to supposedly improve one or more of your executive functions (like working memory).

- *Does the source have a social, political, or other agenda?* Check out its mission statement on the website. Also do an Internet search on the organization to find out what others have to say—often a better way to unveil a hidden agenda. For instance, many people do not realize that the Citizens Commission on Human Rights and their website are a political advocacy arm of the Church of Scientology. Having an agenda doesn't mean the source's information isn't reliable; it just means that overall its message might not be objective.

- *What's the size, scope, and history of the source?* A large national or international organization that has been around for years is generally more reliable than smaller, narrower, and newer ones because a track record of reliable information gathers loyal followers across population sectors—as well as funding.

- *Is the source associated with a center of scientific research?* Sources like the National Institute of Mental Health and major research universities are not just passing on research evidence; they're collecting it. This makes them a *primary* source of information, meaning the data have not been subjected to errors or bias or pulled out of context by *secondary* and more distant sources that have adopted it for their own purposes (however well intentioned).

> Don't forget to educate anyone in a position to help you—spouse, family, friends. A common knowledge base can help all of you cope more effectively and establish realistic goals and expectations.

To find reliable, up-to-date information on the best possible treatments, search the Internet for **consensus guidelines,** promulgated by large, well-respected associations like the World Federation of ADHD, and for **evidence-based treatments**—a slightly more politically tinged and variable term but an attempt by various bodies to establish criteria for treatments supported by the greatest amount of reliable research evidence.

A **randomized, controlled, double-blind trial** is considered the most reliable way to test the effects of a treatment—medication, psychotherapy, or others—because:

- The study subjects are divided into two groups at **random,** meaning by chance. This reduces the opportunity for bias in choosing who gets what treatment or a placebo. As a result, the results are more likely to be due to the treatment, if effective, than to some other confounding variable or factor.

- The population sample is reasonably large and recruited from a variety of sources, so the study results could be said to be representative of a wide range of individuals.

- The effects that might be seen for the treatment under scrutiny are **controlled** by having one of the groups receive only a placebo (non-active "fake" treatment, like a sugar pill), so there's a way to compare. (When scientists give everyone in a group a placebo, roughly a third of them will say they got the effect that the active treatment was supposed to produce! This is called the *placebo effect.*)

- The study is **double-blind,** meaning there's no chance of the researchers projecting their own bias onto their observations because neither the study coordinator nor the study subjects know who's getting the active treatment and who's getting the placebo.

Look closely at the content of the claims:

- *Does the claim sound too good to be true?* It probably is. If ADHD were caused by easily modified dietary habits or could be erased for good by a pill or a machine, would millions of adults and kids still have the condition?

- *Does it include hard facts and figures?* General terms like *most, many, hardly ever, few, experts agree, everyone knows, clinical studies* (a fancy name used in ads for "we gave it to people and they said it worked fine"), and *doctors say* can cover up a void in real research data. If the material fails to give numbers, facts, and names, the claims probably aren't based on any.

- *Are references listed?* A wealth of references on which the claims are based can offset a lack of data in the text; some reliable sources try to make the take-home messages easy to absorb and then trust you to look up the original research. Do a spot-check of such references just to make sure they're real even if you've decided the source is trustworthy and the general points are all you need.

- *How much evidence is there?* Have the research studies been repeated at a number of labs with similar results? Is the evidence mainly "anecdotal," meaning it comes from clinical practice (reports of practitioners from their observations of patients)? It's better when it comes from formal lab studies, with the 24-karat variety being "randomized, controlled, double-blind trials," but keep in mind that research is expensive to fund, and many worthy treatments start out with tons of clinical evidence to support them before they undergo a look in the lab to confirm their findings. It's also helpful to know when the same evidence keeps turning up over the years, and studies of the same population over many years—called *longitudinal studies*—are the only way to be sure what effects a medication or other therapy will have years later, whether you've continued taking it or not.

A Twist of Facts

In early 2008 I was interviewed for a *New York Times* article* reporting on a groundbreaking study by the National Institute of Mental Health: Brain-imaging technology graphically showed that kids with ADHD experience a delay in the development of parts of the brain that affect executive functions like paying attention and memory. At last we had proof of a biological basis for ADHD. Surely those who had argued for years that ADHD did not exist would be enlightened. Imagine the surprise of the NIMH investigators and many other scientists, like me, when instead this evidence was offered as proof of the opposite—that ADHD was "merely" a delay and that kids with the symptoms were normal and would outgrow them. We know from many studies that possibly only a third of children who qualify for the diagnosis no longer qualify for it by adulthood. **When you read about research evidence, make sure you know what data the research produced and what conclusions the scientists drew (such as using Google Scholar). Conclusions drawn by other parties, especially nonscientists, particularly when they disagree with the analysis of the investigators, are questionable.**

---

*"Attention Deficits That May Linger Well Past Childhood," by Aliyah Baruchin, *New York Times*, March 13, 2008.

Step Three

Change Your Brain

Medications for Mastering ADHD

Here are some good reasons to consider medication:

- The professional who evaluated you concluded that you have moderate to severe ADHD.

- Research shows medications are the most effective treatment currently available for ADHD, being at least twice as effective as nonmedication treatments like counseling or behavior therapy and improving symptoms in 70–95% of the adults who take them.

- You've tried other therapies and your symptoms are still causing the same problems they always have.

- You have to do a lot of work independently and can't depend on others to routinely structure your work or home life for you.

- You're having trouble performing well amid all the distractions and pressures of your workplace.

- Your workplace evaluations from your supervisors are increasingly negative or critical, and you sense you may be on the verge of being laid off or fired.

- Your time management is far poorer than that of your typical peers: You are chronically late with deadlines, have lots of missed appointments or meetings, cannot seem to pay your bills on time, and are frequently late to work.

- You've repeatedly tried to finish your education but can never seem to get those last few credits completed, projects done, or other class requirements met that would allow you to graduate.

- You're tired of spending half your life on damage control and want to stop feeling demoralized by not having accomplished much of what you had hoped to achieve by this point.

- You've been diagnosed not only with ADHD but also with anxiety, depression, or another mental or emotional condition.

- Your spouse or someone you're dating is considering separating from you because of your ADHD symptoms, your problems with emotional self-control, and their impact on your relationship.

- Others repeatedly tell you how poor your driving is or how many risks you take on the road. Maybe you're in danger of losing your license because of multiple speeding or parking tickets.

- You have a hard time managing your money, and you know you spend too much or you use your credit cards more than you really want to.

- You've noticed that your health is not as good as that of others. Maybe you have harmful habits you'd like to get rid of, like smoking, drinking too much, eating poorly and too much, or not exercising enough, but you can't seem to kick them.

12

Why It Makes Sense
to Try Medication*

Medication works.

When people ask why they should try medication as a way to manage their ADHD, my answer always comes down to those two words. That's because ADHD medications are the most effective treatments currently available for mastering your ADHD. Period.

> We now know that ADHD medications can *normalize* the behavior of 50–65% of those with ADHD and result in *substantial improvements,* if not normalization, in another 20–30% of people with the disorder.

When you find the medicine that is right for you, you can experience substantial improvements in your ADHD symptoms. Once you do, you can expect significant improvements in the impairments caused by those symptoms. In fact, the positive change brought about by ADHD medications is probably unrivaled by any medication treatment for any other disorder in psychiatry.

---

*Dr. Barkley has worked as a paid consultant to and/or speaker for Eli Lilly (United States, Canada, Spain, Italy, the Netherlands, Sweden, the United Kingdom, Germany), Shire Pharmaceuticals (now Takeda Pharmaceutical Co.; United States), Novartis (United States, Switzerland, Germany), Ortho-McNeil (United States), Janssen-Ortho (Canada), Janssen-Cilag (Denmark, the Netherlands, South America), Ironshore Pharmaceuticals and Development (United States), and Medice Pharma Co. (Germany and Switzerland).

Why Are These Medications So Effective?

Research over the last decade has shown that these medications actually correct or compensate for the neurological problems underlying ADHD. They do so temporarily, only as long as they are in your bloodstream and brain, which means you have to keep taking them to keep getting their benefits.

● ● ● ● ● ● ● ● ● ● ● ● ● ● ● ● ● ●

Fewer than 10% of people with ADHD will *not* have a positive response to at least one of the ADHD medications currently available in the United States.

● ● ● ● ● ● ● ● ● ● ● ● ● ● ● ● ● ●

Here's how the anti-ADHD medications work neurogenetically:

Brain imaging, EEGs, and a variety of other testing methods have shown that the brains of those with ADHD are different from those of others in several important ways:

● Certain regions of the brain are different structurally, mainly being smaller than in those without ADHD: the prefrontal region, associated with attention and inhibition; the striatal region, associated with pursuing pleasurable or rewarding behavior; the anterior cingulate cortex, which helps you with choices among conflicting actions and consequences, as well as with self-regulating your emotional reactions; and the cerebellum, associated with the timing and timeliness of your actions, as well as the fluidity or gracefulness of those actions, among other executive functions. In children and teens with ADHD these brain regions are 2–3 years behind in their maturation.

● Studies show that the white-matter fiber bundles in the brain that connect various brain regions and coordinate their functions are less well developed, less well connected, and highly variable in their activity. This is particularly true for the frontal–striatal–cerebellar executive circuits.

● People with ADHD have less electrical activity in the brain, particularly in those regions noted just above, and are less responsive to events, meaning they don't react to stimulation of these regions as much as others do.

• Children and adolescents with ADHD may also have less metabolic activity in certain frontal regions.

• The brains of those with ADHD seem to be deficient in or show excessive reuptake of norepinephrine and dopamine in certain regions related to attention, inhibition, and executive functioning. Other neurochemicals may also be involved.

Scientists believe the structural abnormalities in the ADHD brain and their poor functional connectivity likely underlie the development of the disorder. This is the genetic legacy that causes most ADHD cases and accounts for why it appears in the descendants of those who have ADHD. In others, the disorder may arise from injuries to these brain areas, such as from exposure to prenatal toxins, premature birth, or repeated head trauma during development. We don't know how to restore a typical structure to these brains.

We do, however, know how to correct the neurochemical imbalances and functional irregularities found in those with ADHD, at least temporarily: medication.

When the neurotransmitters dopamine and norepinephrine are not available in the same measure as they are in typical adults, the messages these chemicals are supposed to send don't get through as they should. Without the help of these neurotransmitters, the brain does not respond to stimulation (any input, like an event or an idea or an emotion) the way it should. Impulse control doesn't kick in when it should. Memories of the past and visions of the future aren't triggered and held in working memory to keep you mentally on track. And even when they are, they cannot be sustained for very long, leading you to forget what it is you were planning on doing. The motor-control brakes don't keep you from fidgeting with restlessness.

This is why ADHD medications work (though some operate on other neurochemicals). By causing nerve cells to express more of these neurochemicals, keeping the nerve cells from pulling them back in once they've been released, or reducing "noise" in the nerve signal, they increase communication between nerve cells in regions of the brain linked to ADHD. The three basic categories of drugs approved by the U.S. Food and Drug Administration for use with adults who have ADHD—stimulants, nonstimulants, and alpha-2 hypertension drugs—boost your mind's ability to respond to whatever is going on in your day. They don't all work the same way, but the end result is that they manage the symptoms of ADHD effectively in most cases.

Check the resources starting on page 278 for updates on how the ADHD medications work within the brain, right down to how the medications affect the functioning of nerve cells. We're learning more every day. Studies in molecular genetics also help explain and predict the improvements you're likely to experience from these medicines.

The beauty of what we know about how the medications work is that it proves they are not simply masking or covering up the symptoms of ADHD, and it confirms our knowledge about the functioning of the brain regions involved and its connection to these symptoms. These medicines are not "Band-Aids," "billy clubs," "chemical straitjackets," or merely "mother's little helpers," as some critics in the popular media have contended. *While active in your body, they correct or compensate for the biological problem at the bottom of ADHD.*

If you've been exposed to claims that these medications just cover up what's wrong, you might have doubts about trying them. I hope this chapter will eliminate your concerns. Opting not to use medication to master your ADHD, for whatever reason, means denying yourself the most effective treatment currently available. It's like a diabetic choosing not to use insulin but instead trying to deal with the diabetes strictly through diet and more exercise. Maybe that will work, but it's less likely to do so and will result in far less control of the disorder than using medication to manage it. Why would you deny yourself the equivalent of insulin for a diabetic?

The effectiveness of medication doesn't mean it's the only treatment available. If your symptoms are mild, you may get what you need from the strategies and tools in Steps Four and Five or from a special form of cognitive-behavioral therapy that targets your executive function deficits. Coaching might be of great benefit. Support groups could provide you with shared ideas and inspiration. But if your symptoms are moderate to severe, medication can alleviate a lot of your struggles and allow you to get much more out of the nonmedication help available.

Also, if being evaluated for ADHD has revealed that you have more than one disorder to deal with, you could benefit from medications that can address all your problems. Studies have shown that sometimes anxiety and depression are caused by the difficulties of living with ADHD and that when ADHD symptoms are alleviated through medication, anxiety and depression recede.

As with most conditions, mental or physical, the symptoms occur along a continuum from mildest to most severe. This is why diagnostic criteria are important. Health professionals do not want to treat people unnecessarily. If you have some symptoms, but not enough to meet the DSM criteria, and you are experiencing impairment in certain major life activities, you will be said to have *subclinical* ADHD, sometimes called ADHD NOS (NOS = *not otherwise specified*). *In that case medication may or may not be prescribed,* even if ADHD medication was

In my book *ADHD in Adults: What the Science Says,* my coauthors and I compared adults with ADHD who had been diagnosed as children with those who had been diagnosed as adults. We looked at the data collected in our Milwaukee study, which followed children from the late 1970s into adulthood in the new millennium, and also the data collected in a University of Massachusetts Medical Center study of adults.

- We found remarkable similarities between the two groups. The evidence showed that at least half of the children diagnosed with ADHD still met the criteria for the disorder as adults.

- Those diagnosed as adults tended to be less impaired than those diagnosed as children and followed to adulthood.

- But 85% of those diagnosed as adults were more likely to have other disorders too, particularly anxiety and depression. Why? We don't know for sure, but it could be that anxiety and depression were the result of having struggled with ADHD symptoms for years without treatment.

- Those diagnosed as kids had greater problems with educational and occupational performance, and a substantial minority had more antisocial behavior and drug use. Again, why? Perhaps these individuals were diagnosed early in life because their impairments were more noticeable, suggesting their symptoms may have been more severe than the symptoms of those who made it through to adulthood before getting diagnosed.

What this means regarding medication for adults with ADHD:

- *If you were diagnosed recently,* you may need other medications besides those for ADHD to ensure that you get help for anxiety or depression along with ADHD.

- *If you were diagnosed as a child,* you may need ADHD medication again if your symptoms are moderate to severe and you are experiencing impairment in one or more major life activities.

prescribed for you when you were a child. Even so, if impairment exists, ask for the medicine even if you are a symptom or two shy of the diagnosis.

If your attitude about trying medication is tied up with emotions and self-image, a therapist or other counselor may be able to help you examine whether these issues should factor into your treatment decisions. In the meantime, keep asking yourself this essential question:

> "Do I deserve to have a tougher life than other people just because I was born with a biological predisposition to ADHD?"

I don't know too many people whose answer would be "yes."

If you've never taken medication for ADHD, do you have doubts about starting?

- Maybe you've just been diagnosed, and treatment options never entered your mind before now.

- Maybe being handed a prescription would make the disorder all too real for you, and you're not quite ready to own ADHD, as discussed in Chapter 11.

- Are you afraid of becoming "dependent" on a drug?

- Do you subscribe to the notion that not managing your symptoms on your own is a sign of weakness?

What Medication Choices Do I Have?

Many. The medications proven effective for treating ADHD fall into three groups: the stimulants (methylphenidate, amphetamine), the nonstimulants (atomoxetine and viloxazine), and the alpha-2 antihypertensive medicines guanfacine XR (XR means "extended release") and clonidine XR. The information that follows should help you understand the recommendations your doctor might make. It will also help you make the treatment decisions that are right for you.

You probably have lots of questions—about how to take the medications, about their safety and effectiveness, about any side effects that you should expect, and more. Fortunately, thousands of adults with ADHD before you have asked the same questions. And physicians and therapists all over the world have had decades of experience in answering them. Chapters 13 and 14—and Chapter 15, which tells you what to expect from a course of treatment from beginning to end—give you the benefit of that experience.

My Position on ADHD Medications

- ADHD is a disabling condition that arises from neurological and genetic factors and causes problems in every area of life. Using a medication to manage a neurogenetic disorder is perfectly reasonable and not just a means of covering up the "real" social or personal causes of your symptoms. ADHD does not arise from social factors or mere personal choices. You deserve to reap the benefits of any treatment **proven** to help.

- You should **not** be prescribed medication for ADHD without a firm diagnosis following a thorough evaluation by a qualified mental health professional.

- Myths about ADHD medications abound. Quantity does not equal quality. You can and should get the facts from your doctor and other reliable sources (see Chapter 11).

- No prescription treatment is etched in stone. You can try a different medication or stop medication altogether if it proves ineffective or produces intolerable side effects.

- Medication should always be prescribed as a collaborative effort between you and your physician.

The table here sums up the medications currently available and FDA approved for adult ADHD, the forms they come in, and how long their effects last after a dose. This is a handy reference you might end up coming back to again and again.

Generic name (brand name)	Duration of activity	How supplied
MPH (Ritalin)[a]	3–4 hours	Tablets (5, 10, 20 mg)
d-MPH (Focalin)[a]	3–4 hours	Tablets (2.5, 5, 10 mg; 2.5 mg Focalin equivalent to 5 mg Ritalin)
MPH (Methylin)[a]	3–4 hours	Tablets (5, 10, 20 mg)
MPH SR (Ritalin SR)[a]	3–8 hours (variable)	Tablets (20 mg; amount absorbed appears to vary)

(cont.)

Generic name (brand name)	Duration of activity	How supplied
MPH (Metadate ER)[a]	3–8 hours (variable)	Tablets (10, 20 mg; amount absorbed appears to vary)
MPH (Methylin ER)[a]	8 hours	Tablets (10, 20 mg); chewable tablets (2.5, 5, 10 mg); oral solution (5 mg/5 ml, 10 mg/5 ml)
MPH (Ritalin LA)[a]	8 hours	Capsules (20, 30, 40 mg; can be sprinkled)
MPH (Metadate CD)[a]	8 hours	Capsules (20 mg; can be sprinkled)
MPH (Concerta)[a]	12 hours	Caplets (18, 27, 36, 54 mg)
d-MPH XR (Focalin XR)[a,c]	12 hours	Capsules (10, 20, 30 mg)
AMP (Dexedrine)[b]	4–5 hours	Tablets (5 mg)
AMP (Dextrostat)[b]	4–5 hours	Tablets (5, 10 mg)
AMP (Dexedrine Spansules)[b]	8 hours	Capsules (5, 10, 15 mg)
Mixed salts of AMP (Adderall)[b]	4–6 hours	Tablets (5, 7.5, 10, 12.5, 15, 20, 30 mg)
Mixed salts of AMP (Adderall XR)[a,c]	At least 8 hours (but appears to last much longer in certain patients)	Capsules (5, 10, 15, 20, 25, 30 mg; can be sprinkled)
lisdexamfetamine dimesylate (Vyvanse)[c]	At least 8 hours (but appears to last much longer in certain patients)	Capsules (20, 30, 40, 50, 60, 70 mg)
atomoxetine (Strattera)[a,c]	8–10 hours or more (5-hour plasma half-life but much longer in central nervous system)	Capsules (10, 18, 25, 40, 60, 80 mg)
viloxazine (Qelbree)	At least 8–9 hours (7-hour half-life)	Capsules (100, 150, 200 mg)
guanfacine XR (Intuniv)[a,c]	24 hours	Tablets (1, 2, 3, 4 mg)
clonidine XR (Kapvay)	24 hours	Tablets (1 mg)

Note. MPH: methylphenidate; AMP: amphetamine.

[a]Approved to treat ADHD in patients age 6 years and older.
[b]Approved to treat ADHD in patients age 3 years and older.
[c]Specifically approved for treatment of ADHD in adults.

13

The Stimulants

The stimulants are the ADHD medications you're most likely to have heard of. They've been around longest and are used for both kids and adults. If you were diagnosed as a child, a stimulant might have been recommended as part of your treatment years ago. Stimulants are also the most controversial medications for ADHD. That is because unlike the nonstimulants, they are classified as Schedule II (potentially addictive) medications by the Drug Enforcement Administration. Despite that classification, when they are taken orally as prescribed for ADHD the risk for addiction is low to nonsignificant. Myths as well as realistic concerns appear regularly in the news, however, and fly about the Internet pretty constantly. This chapter will:

✓ Sort fact from fiction

✓ Give you an idea of whether a stimulant might help you

✓ Answer the questions typically raised about these medications by adults with ADHD

The Stimulants: Pros and Cons

The Pros: The stimulants increase inhibition, resistance to distraction, and the capacity to sustain attention while holding in mind what you are supposed to be doing or planning to do. They increase motor timing and coordination as well as emotional self-control. As a result, they reduce the adverse impact these and other ADHD symptoms have on various domains of our major life activities. With the new sustained-release forms of these medicines, these positive benefits can last for 8–12 hours instead of the 3–5 that are typical with immediate-release forms.

The Cons: Some people experience problems with insomnia, loss of appetite, stomachaches, and headaches with these medications. Others feel somewhat tense, as if they have had too much caffeine, for instance. A small percentage of cases report increased anxiety, tics, or other nervous mannerisms, especially if these were problems that existed before starting medications. The medicines cannot be taken 24 hours a day, so they can leave some times of the day uncovered or with too little medication for it to be effective, such as late evening hours if the medicine was taken in the morning.

How Do Stimulants Help?

Two basic types of stimulants are currently marketed in the United States: methylphenidate (MPH) and amphetamine (AMP). But they come in a variety of delivery systems that determine how long they will remain in the body and actively controlling ADHD symptoms.

Generic name	Brand name	Generic name	Brand name
Methylphenidate	Ritalin	Amphetamine	Dexedrine
	Focalin		Dextrostat
	Methylin		Adderall
	Metadate		Vyvanse
	Concerta		

Note. A third stimulant, pemoline (brand name Cylert), was available for nearly 30 years but was discontinued due to rare but significant risks for liver damage.

The stimulants help ease ADHD symptoms by increasing the availability of several neurochemicals that carry self-control-boosting messages in the brain, especially dopamine. To be available as messengers, the neurochemicals have to be available in the spaces between nerve cells. Think of them as the water in a system of canals. The amphetamines mainly increase the amount of dopamine (and, to a lesser extent, norepinephrine) produced and expressed by the nerve cells so that more ends up in those spaces. Their effect in the brain is like opening a gate to let the water rush out into the canal. Methylphenidate works differently, by mainly decreasing the amount of dopamine that is reabsorbed into the nerve cell after being released—it keeps the lock closed so that the water (neurochemical) level remains high in the canal once it has been released there.

 Why wouldn't an ADHD medicine like the stimulants make me even more antsy than I already am?

The term *stimulant* is misleading. Stimulant medications like methylphenidate (Ritalin and the like) do make people without ADHD more alert and awake;

Why are the stimulants frequently abused? In those who have typical levels of dopamine in the brain, the boost afforded by the stimulants provides a pleasant sensation of "speediness." But that's not all. The stimulants increase dopamine in the regions of the brain known to increase the likelihood of drug addiction (the reward center, or nucleus acumbens)—some of the same regions where the drugs do so much good for people with ADHD. This activates the brain's reward centers, determining how pleasurable or reinforcing certain stimuli will be. The increased activity in these centers can result in increased sensations of euphoria, interest, or other reward-related experiences. These pleasurable altered states of consciousness are most likely to occur when stimulants are taken intravenously or snorted into the sinus passages as a powder, allowing the drug to enter into and then clear from these brain regions rapidly. It is this rapid alteration in conscious sensations that creates the euphoria or other pleasurable sensations and seems to determine the addictive properties of a medicine.

Why don't adults (or children) with ADHD get hooked on the stimulants? Mainly because the drugs are taken orally, in pill or capsule form, in relatively low doses and thus enter and leave the brain very slowly. Most people who abuse stimulants use higher doses and snort them or inject them into a vein in a solution, such as the stimulant mixed with water. With those delivery systems the drugs hit the brain all at once with a much more powerful wallop. Also, when these medications are used to treat ADHD they are only bringing the dopamine levels up to normal, not raising them rapidly well above normal levels as they would in someone attempting to abuse the drugs through intranasal or intravenous use.

they stimulate activity in the frontal regions of the brain, improving inhibition, sustained attention, and other executive functions necessary for typical self-regulation. The reason they don't make hyperactive kids and adults even more restless than they already are due to ADHD is that these parts of the brain are underactive or underreactive in those with ADHD. There's not enough norepinephrine and dopamine available to send signals between neurons and stimulate the mind to do what it's supposed to do—pay attention, sit still, look before leaping, and so forth.

While stimulants can also stimulate the brain to do what it's supposed to do in typical adults, the degree of improvement is far less dramatic than in those with ADHD. This is most likely due to the marked underfunctioning of these brain regions in those with ADHD that is not evident in a typical brain.

Are the Stimulants Safe?

Yes! Very safe. But obviously, the stimulants can be abused by anyone. That's why they are classified as Schedule II and *potentially* addictive controlled substances. Through this classification the U.S. government puts strict limits on the amounts of these drugs that manufacturers can produce every year, on how they can be prescribed, and on how pharmacies store and dispense them. It also means if you decide to try them, you need to take responsibility for keeping them locked up in a safe place where no one but you can get them.

But what about the potential danger to you? You may have heard a couple of different myths about the stimulants. It's time to set the story straight:

Do the Stimulants Lead to Abuse of Other Drugs?

You may have heard claims that these drugs increase the sensitivity to or risk for abusing other drugs, especially other stimulants. The vast majority of research does not support this claim. More than 16 studies have examined this issue, many, like my own, having followed children with ADHD treated with stimulants for months or years into adulthood. They did not find any increase in risk for later drug abuse. Evidence for claims that these drugs can sensitize the brain, making later exposure to stimulants more powerful and potentially addicting, comes only from studies of animals in which the drugs were given intravenously, injected directly into the brain, or given in much higher doses than is the case when treating children or adults with ADHD. So, the evidence to date does not support any claims that using stimulants as prescribed for managing ADHD contributes to the risk of abusing these or other drugs now or later in life.

Do the Stimulants Cause Heart Attacks or Strokes?

You may have heard that these drugs can increase the risk of sudden death, usually from heart block, and that people taking stimulants have, even more rarely, suffered strokes. Sudden deaths that occur when the heart stops beating have all been traced to other factors, like a history of structural heart defects along with vigorous exercise right before the death or a family (genetic) history of sudden death. These factors alone can account for sudden death. The available evidence actually shows that people on stimulants have a somewhat lower likelihood of sudden death than the general population. This is probably because physicians routinely screen for heart problems before prescribing stimulants and don't use them for anyone with a family history of sudden death or a personal history of structural heart abnormalities, major arrhythmias, other major cardiac problems, or even high blood pressure. This means that those at greatest cardiac risk with stimulants usually don't end up with this prescription. This could be why the risk ends up *lower* than in the general population.

> **The stimulants increase heart rate and blood pressure, but only as much as climbing a half flight of stairs. There's no evidence that they cause high blood pressure in those who didn't already have it.**

> Research shows that sudden death occurs in one to three of 100,000 people taking stimulants for ADHD every year, versus one to seven out of every 100,000 in the general population. So the rate of sudden death in those taking stimulants is not significantly higher than that for the general population that is not taking stimulants. In fact, it was somewhat lower in this research. That's because people about to take a stimulant prescription get a physical exam and screen for possible cardiac problems. When cardiac problems are detected, they are typically not prescribed stimulants. This is not the case for the general population, which is not being routinely screened for heart problems.

How long can I continue to take a stimulant without any long-term negative effects?

As far as we know, you can take it for as many years as you may need to manage your symptoms and reduce related impairments.

Is there any scientific evidence to suggest that Ritalin or other stimulant medication is either safe or unsafe during pregnancy?

There is now a small amount of evidence concerning the effects of ADHD medications on pregnant mothers or their babies, but no evidence of major abnormalities in babies born to mothers who stayed on their ADHD medication. There is some research showing that small amounts of amphetamine may enter the mother's breast milk and thus her newborn if she is breastfeeding, but not enough to harm the infant. This does not seem to occur with methylphenidate (Ritalin and the like). But because the amount of available evidence is still small, at this time all companies recommend that women discontinue their ADHD medications should they become pregnant. Keep in mind that this advice is based to some extent on companies wishing to limit their liability, not just on the prevailing evidence.

There are numerous risks to coming off medication and allowing one's ADHD to go back to its high, unmanaged levels, including an increase in the risk of accidental injuries, car crashes, abuse of other drugs, suicide, earlier death (from those risks), and overeating, as well as greater loss of emotional control and adverse effects on parenting. These risks must be weighed against any hypothetical risk to the baby from a parent continuing on medication while pregnant.

What Side Effects Can I Expect?

These are the most common side effects adults experience when taking a stimulant, from most to least common:

✓ Insomnia

✓ Loss of appetite

✓ Weight loss

✓ Headaches

✓ Nausea, upset stomach, or stomachache

✓ Anxiety

✓ Irritability

✓ Motor tics

✓ Increased muscle tension

You can find a simple list like this in the package insert that comes with your prescription. That doesn't tell you much about the impact you can really expect the stimulants to have on your daily life. These firsthand reports illustrate both what you might experience and how to counteract any negative effects:

"I had never been treated for my ADHD before, always believing that the symptoms were really just a reflection of my own personal failings or lack of self-discipline. But when my doctor started me on a stimulant for my ADHD, the results amazed me. I actually could remember multiple things in my mind that I needed to do without losing them to the nearest distractions. And I was able to persist at work I usually found boring far longer than before, which meant I was much more productive at getting things done, and done more quickly and efficiently, because I could focus better on the tasks at hand. I know it sounds weird, but I could actually see things more clearly—not so much things around me, but the ideas I was holding in my mind about what I wanted to do were more clear, less jumbled and disorganized, and more likely to lead me to get them done.

"I did have less of an appetite, particularly for midday meals, but I had been meaning to drop a few pounds anyway, so that was no big deal. And I did find myself staying up a little later at night before falling asleep, but not so much that it affected me the next day. Overall, being treated for my ADHD has literally saved my job and my marriage. At times I still need some help with structuring my work late in the day, especially when the medicine may be wearing off. But on balance this treatment has helped me turn my life around."

"I took Ritalin in second and third grade, and it made me really jittery and nervous. I didn't want to go to school for a long time. I felt a little calmer once the doctor took me off it. But then I didn't want to go to school because I couldn't sit still and concentrate! I still have anxiety today, so I wasn't too eager to take the Adderall my doctor suggested recently. But she prescribed an antianxiety drug along with the Adderall, and they've worked great for me."

The research is somewhat mixed on whether stimulants worsen anxiety, but enough studies have found this to be the case (though more with children than adults and more with amphetamines than methylphenidate) that you should be aware of this possible adverse effect. If you are concerned about anxiety, the nonstimulants might be a better choice (see Chapter 14).

"Yeah, sometimes I have a really hard time falling asleep at night. But I drink warm milk, and a friend taught me deep breathing and progressive relaxation, and that often helps. On an up note, I've lost that 10 pounds I could never shed: these days I never seem to want lunch, maybe because the stimulant is at its peak in my system then, and I think I'm just eating the right number of calories now."

"When my brother started taking a stimulant, he said all of a sudden he was snapping at people and losing his temper all the time. His doctor reduced the dosage, and he felt better, although he didn't get the same amount of help with his ADHD symptoms that way. But when I took the same medicine, I felt pretty calm, like I could control my emotions for the first time in I don't know how long."

In rare cases, stimulants make people more irritable or angry, most often later in the day when the medicine might be wearing off. A few report feelings of mild sadness or emotional sensitivity that can make them prone to tearfulness. But such effects are rare and dissipate within hours of discontinuing the medicine. Whether stimulants are likely to make you feel this way may depend on your own personality, what other disorders you may have along with your ADHD, and which of your executive functions have been affected most by ADHD. If you had a lot of trouble controlling your emotions in the past, and you haven't been diagnosed with a problem like depression in addition to ADHD, the stimulants may actually improve your emotional self-control. Emotion regulation is one of the executive functions weakened by ADHD and improved by medication treatment.

"When they first started working, these medications made me feel like my whole body was tense—like I might be clenching my jaw and grinding my teeth—and I was always on the verge of a headache. Sometimes my back felt really tight too. It was like I'd had four cups of coffee instead of my usual one or two. My doctor reduced my dosage slightly. Also, now I go to the gym and work out, which makes me at least feel more relaxed before I get home from work. My wife says I've not only trimmed down but bulked up my muscles too."

Actual increases in muscle tension are not common side effects of stimulant treatment. More often it is a subjective feeling of tenseness but even that is uncommon. Yet some people do experience them, especially if they are taking higher-than-typical doses. This is more likely to happen on an amphetamine than on methylphenidate. Unless you have a family history of tic disorders or previously had them yourself, the stimulants are unlikely to cause motor tics. If you have a family or personal history, you might develop them while on stimulants. Up to a third of those who already have tics will see them worsen. But another third found no increase in tics, and a third of those who had a tic disorder previously have actually reported some improvement. Therefore, a personal or family history of tic disorders should not preclude trying a stimulant—you only need to be extra vigilant about monitoring for the occurrence of tics to evaluate how the drug may be affecting them.

 This medicine really helps my ADHD symptoms, but it makes me really nauseated. What can I do?

This can happen if you take the medicine on an empty stomach, so try eating something before you take your medication. If the problem continues, speak with your doctor about reducing the dose, changing the time you take the dose, or switching to another medication.

 Can I drink alcohol or take other drugs when I am on a stimulant for ADHD management?

Yes, but you should do so in moderation. The only drugs you should avoid, of course, are other stimulants, such as cocaine, methamphetamine, crack, or another prescription stimulant, as this just increases the effect of the other stimulant on your body. But caffeine and alcohol do not interact adversely with the stimulants. Nicotine can act as a stimulant, compounding the effects of your ADHD medicines on your heart rate and blood pressure. Please discuss this with your doctor if you are a smoker.

What Are My Choices?

The stimulants come in different forms or delivery systems: *pills* (tablets), *pumps* (capsules), *pellets* (capsules and caplets), *patches*, and *pro-drug* (capsules). For children, there are also delayed activation, liquid, and oral dissolving (gummy) formulations.

Look for these brand names for stimulants in pill form:

- Ritalin (MPH, a mixture of d-MPH and l-MPH)
- Focalin (just d-MPH)
- Dexedrine (d-AMP)
- Adderall and Evekeo are both mixtures of l- and d-AMP.

. . . .
Your choice of drug form will depend largely on what matters to you, like how long your active day is and when you need to be on top of your game. All of these delivery systems have been proven safe and effective in hundreds of studies.
. . . .

Pills

These are the original versions of these medicines, and they've been available for many decades. The first versions of amphetamine were developed in the 1930s, while the first version of methylphenidate was created in the 1950s. In pill form, these medications are absorbed quickly, usually within 15–20 minutes after being taken by mouth and swallowed. They can usually reach their peak level in the blood (and so in the brain) in 60–90 minutes and may control the symptoms of ADHD for 3–5 hours. That's their main problem. If you want to control the symptoms of ADHD for the typical 14- to 16-hour adult day, you have to take these medications two to four times a day or even more often.

. . . .
Pro: Rapid activation, short duration of action (when the drug is needed for just a short time)
. . . .

. . . .
Con: Need to remember to take the next dose several times a day—probably not one of your strengths.
. . . .

. . . .
Pros:

- 8–12 hours of symptom control from one dose
- Possibly the best time-release form of methylphenidate if you need to be at peak performance in the afternoon
. . . .

The Pump

Then came the invention of an ingenious water-based (osmotic) pump system for delivering these drugs into the body and keeping them in the bloodstream longer. The brand name for this system is Concerta, and it delivers methylphenidate. It's a container that looks like a capsule, with a small laser-drilled hole on one of its long ends. Inside are two chambers. One chamber contains a paste-like sludge of methylphenidate, and the other chamber is empty. There is also a powdered form of methylphenidate that coats the outside of the capsule. Now here is the neat part: When you swallow the capsule, the powder goes right to work just as it would in the pill form. That gets some medication into the bloodstream quickly and gives the capsule just enough time to start to absorb water from your stomach (and later your intestines). The water is absorbed through the wall of the pump in a continuous, even flow into that empty chamber. As that chamber fills up, it presses against the chamber containing the methylphenidate paste and squeezes it out of the hole in the capsule continuously for 8–12 hours or more. The end result is that many people, especially children, need to take only one capsule a day and not the usual two to three (or more) they would have to take using the regular pills.

Cons:

- A standard pill may need to be added to extend symptom control to a full adult day
- Not easy to adjust the dose due to limited capsule sizes

The capsules come in various doses, of course, so your doctor can adjust the dose to suit your individual needs and responses. One problem, though, is that some adults in particular may need a longer course of medication each day than what the capsule provides. To deal with that issue, some physicians prescribe the immediate-release pill form of methylphenidate or amphetamine toward the end of the day to provide an extra 3–5 hours of treatment with medication when the Concerta may be losing its beneficial control of ADHD symptoms. Even so, you just have to love the human ingenuity that led to the discovery of this delivery system.

The Pellets

At around the same time as the water-pump method was being invented, engineers were modifying a method that uses time-release pellets to keep medicines in the body and bloodstream longer than the pills. This method had been used for years with some cold medicines but had to be modified in various ways for use with methylphenidate and amphetamine. Now we have time-release pellets for both of these stimulants. Little beads of the drug are coated in such a way that some dissolve immediately after being swallowed, while others dissolve 1, 2, 3, or more hours later so that the drug can be absorbed more gradually into the bloodstream across 8–10 hours for most people. This ingenious delivery system has the added advantage that anyone who simply cannot or does not want to swallow the capsule containing these pellets can open the capsule (pull it apart), sprinkle

> Look for these stimulant brand names in pellet form:
> - Ritalin LA (MPH)
> - Focalin XR (d-MPH)
> - Metadate CD (MPH)
> - Adderall XR (AMP)

Pros:

- Great for those who can't (or don't want to) swallow a capsule
- May be best for you if you need to be at your peak in the morning

the contents on a teaspoon of applesauce, yogurt, or other food, and swallow it that way. It does not change the way the drug will work in the body.

Again, there are different sizes (doses) of these capsules to permit your physician to adjust the dose to its optimum level for you. Like the water-pump method, these time-release pellet systems sometimes have to be supplemented late in the day with a regular or immediate-release pill version of the same drug if you need longer symptom control than what these systems can provide into the evening hours. Some research shows that this pellet system provides a little better control of ADHD symptoms in the morning than the afternoon hours, while the pump system provides a bit better control in the afternoon.

Con: The pill may be needed to extend symptom control into the evening.

The Patch

The next invention of a delivery system for the stimulants was approved by the FDA in 2007. It is a patch with an adhesive coating that is applied directly to the skin, such as on the back of your shoulder or on the buttocks. The patch, which goes by the brand name Daytrana, contains methylphenidate. When applied this way, the methylphenidate is absorbed through the skin and gets into the bloodstream by that means. So long as you wear the patch, methylphenidate is being delivered to your bloodstream—for as many hours during the day as you want. As with the other drug forms, the patch comes in different doses so you can take the amount that's best for you.

Pros:
- **Symptom control for as long a day as you want**
- **Nothing to swallow**

Cons:
- **Needs to be removed several hours before bedtime to prevent insomnia**
- **Causes skin rash at patch site in 15–20% of people**

The Pro-Drug

In 2008, another delivery system received FDA approval for use by adults with ADHD, and that system goes by the brand name of Vyvanse (an amphetamine). Here is yet another example of human inventiveness.

One of the problems with the immediate-release pills as well as the pellet systems is that they have the potential to be abused, usually by crushing and inhaling the powder from the pills or the beads from the pellet systems or by mixing the powder with water and injecting it into a vein. This problem led a small biotech company to invent a method in which the amphetamine cannot be activated unless it is in the human stomach or

Pros:
- **Little or no potential for abuse**
- **Full day of symptom control**

• • • • • •

**Con: May last
longer than desired
when only a short
duration is wanted**

• • • • • •

intestines. They achieved this by bonding a lysine compound to the dextroamphetamine d-AMP so that it locked up the amphetamine so it could not activate without removing the lysine "lock." This bonding of an active drug to another compound that alters its typical pattern of activation creates a type of medication called a *pro-drug* by the FDA. Once the pro-drug is swallowed, a chemical that occurs naturally in the stomach and intestines (and probably the blood in the intestinal lining) splits the lysine from the d-AMP, allowing the d-AMP to go to work. Typically, the effects of the d-AMP last 10–14 hours.

What's on the Horizon

Although not yet approved for ADHD in adults, a new delivery system became available in June 2019 for use by children and teens with ADHD. It uses methylphenidate but binds it into a unique delivery system that creates a delay in the activation of the medication (brand name Jornay PM). Children take the medicine at 9:00 P.M., and the drug activates reliably about 9 hours later. This form was invented to get around the fact that other forms of stimulants can leave children unmedicated at one of the most stressful times of the day for both parent and child, early morning on school days. The company plans to launch an amphetamine version of this delayed-release system and hopes to obtain FDA approval of both medicines for use with adults who have ADHD.

Other companies are experimenting with a combination of a stimulant (amphetamine) and a norepinephrine reuptake inhibitor (NERI) similar to atomoxetine to see if they can achieve better control of a wider array of ADHD symptoms than occurs from either drug type alone. And still others are studying even more specific NERI medicines for their effectiveness for ADHD. I also expect to see even more medicines being developed to target the aspects of brain functioning adversely affected by the genes we are now finding contribute to ADHD.

Can the generics really be as different as they seemed in my case? The pharmacy I go to switched to generic versions of Ritalin, and the new generic did not work nearly as well. My doctor switched me to the brand-name drug, but do I really need to spend the extra money?

Your doctor was correct to believe there can be a significant difference. The generic medications appear not to be manufactured with the same degree of rigor as the brand-name medications. The generics have been associated with numerous reports of greater variability in controlling symptoms on a day-to-day basis and less success overall in managing symptoms. Should that occur, ask to be transferred back to the brand-name medicine.

Should I change medication every time a new drug comes out, even though my current medication seems to work fine? If I don't try the new medications, whose advertising promises great new benefits, will I be missing out?

Generally, it's not a good idea to chase the latest drug if the one you are taking is successfully managing your ADHD symptoms. However, if side effects are annoying and your doctor believes the newer medication may be less likely to cause problems, it may be worth switching drugs or delivery systems. For instance, some adults report that Adderall XR's faster and more subjectively detectable onset of action may be associated with feelings of increased inner tension. Switching to Vyvanse has helped them with a smoother onset and offset of their medication's effects. Both are amphetamines, yet the delivery system for Vyvanse seems to make a difference in how rapidly the dose is felt.

What do I do if I forget to take my medicine?

As long as it's not past 1:00 or 2:00 P.M., you can probably take the drug without much impact on your sleep. If you have forgotten for the day, just take it the next day. There appear to be no problems with abrupt cessation of the stimulants, most likely because they wash out of your body within 24 hours in most cases when taken as prescribed.

Is it possible to build tolerance to stimulant medicines? If so, how do I avoid this, or how do I handle it once I'm experiencing it?

Actual physical tolerance seems unlikely with the current ADHD medications, but some individuals report that their medication seems less effective 3–6 months after starting their treatment. This usually requires adjusting the dose or, sometimes, changing to a different delivery system or medication. Clinically, we sometimes see people complaining that their medicine isn't working as well as before, but further information shows them going through an unusually stressful or demanding period in their life that may exacerbate their ADHD symptoms and make it more difficult for their usual dose to provide adequate treatment. They may need to temporarily change their dose or address the source of the stress at these times.

Some people adjust their view of themselves once on medication and end up focusing so strongly on areas where they haven't experienced improvement that they start to believe the drug isn't working. They may need to stop the medicine for a few days to remind themselves of the positive effects it has had on them—or to discover whether, in fact, the drug is *not* doing anything for them.

14

The Nonstimulants

When doctors and researchers talk about "the nonstimulants" for ADHD, they are typically talking about atomoxetine or the alpha-2 antihypertensive medicine guanfacine XR. You'll find atomoxetine sold under the brand name Strattera and guanfacine XR under the name Intuniv.

See Chapter 11 for a definition of randomized, controlled, double-blind trials.

The FDA approved atomoxetine for the management of child, teen, and adult ADHD in 2003. It was the first (and is still the only) nonstimulant approved for the treatment of ADHD in adults. At the time it was the first new drug approved for ADHD in more than 25 years. Atomoxetine was studied more than any other ADHD drug before receiving FDA approval, with randomized double-blind studies involving more than 6,000 patients worldwide. Although the stimulants have been used for ADHD much longer, there's no doubt that the safety and efficacy of atomoxetine have been well researched.

Atomoxetine (Strattera)

Interestingly, atomoxetine was explored for years as a possible antidepressant. When its manufacturer abandoned that direction (for reasons unknown to us), the company shelved the drug but much later began to look at it as a treatment for ADHD. The drug prevents norepinephrine from being reabsorbed by the nerve cells once released, thus leaving more of the drug outside the cell to act on other, nearby nerve cells. This makes it a natural for treating a disorder marked by a shortage of that chemical messenger. In Chapter 13 you read that the stimulants target mainly the neurotransmitter dopamine. The fact that atomoxetine targets primarily norepinephrine means that it has a slightly different effect on ADHD symptoms. Even so, some research suggests it may indirectly improve dopamine functioning as well. By affecting a different brain chemical, it may work better than the stimulants for some people. It all depends on where your particular

ADHD neurological deficits lie. We're all biologically unique, especially in the organization and functioning of the brain.

Atomoxetine can be taken once or twice a day, depending on the dosage. Most adults take the drug once a day. Its effects last most of the day, so there is no need for an extended-release form for daily coverage, as there is with the stimulants. Most people start by taking the drug in the morning, but if they experience significant drowsiness or tiredness that lasts longer than a few weeks, it may be best to take it at night or to split the dose and take it twice daily. It might take longer for your doctor to arrive at the right dosage for you than it does with the stimulants, however. Your body will take longer to adjust to the side effects of drugs like atomoxetine than to the stimulants. So your doctor will probably want to leave you on a particular dose a bit longer before adjusting it than would be the case with a stimulant.

How Effective Is Atomoxetine Compared to Stimulants?

- On average about 75% of people get positive effects from the stimulants or the nonstimulants.

- Some studies suggest that while 50% of people respond positively to both types of medications, 25% may respond better to a stimulant than to atomoxetine, while the remaining 25% may respond better to atomoxetine than to one of the stimulants.

I heard that this drug takes longer to work than the stimulants. Is that so? If so, how long?

Yes, with atomoxetine it can take 2–4 weeks of gradual dose adjustment before your doctor finds the best level for you. The dose is adjusted more slowly mainly because taking a drug like this one that increases norepinephrine can result in annoying side effects like nausea and drowsiness if the dose is raised too much or too quickly. Another drug that works like atomoxetine (viloxazine, or Qelbree) was FDA approved in April 2021 for use with children and may take less time to adjust to an ideal dose. It may be approved for adults sometime soon. I recommend that adults just starting atomoxetine be patient. You've been dealing with ADHD for years, so a few weeks to achieve good control of your symptoms is a small price to pay for the advantages this drug can provide.

Why Atomoxetine Is Rarely Abused . . . and What This Means to You

Some research shows that by blocking the reuptake of norepinephrine atomoxetine also increases the amount of dopamine outside of nerve cells. But it does so *only in certain parts of the brain, such as the frontal cortex.* This means the drug can address dopamine-related ADHD deficits in the brain *without* affecting the brain reward centers likely to be related to drug addiction or abuse. Because it doesn't have the same stimulant effect as methylphenidate and amphetamine, the drug has little appeal as a drug of abuse. In fact, research shows that people addicted to drugs don't favor atomoxetine any more than they do other psychiatric drugs, such as antidepressants—which is to say very little. This is why it's called a "nonstimulant" and why it's not a controlled substance in the United States.

What does this mean for you?

- It's much more convenient to fill and refill a prescription. Your doctor can phone in a refill, for example, which can't be done with the stimulants.

- You don't have to take the same precautions to keep the drug inaccessible to everyone else.

- This might be the treatment of choice for you if you've struggled with substance abuse of your own. (In fact, one study of adult alcoholics with ADHD showed that atomoxetine improved ADHD and reduced heavy drinking at the same time.)

Is Atomoxetine Safe?

✓ It's certainly safe in terms of its abuse potential—it has none.

✓ Liver complications occur once in every million people treated—one to four cases out of 4.5 million treated at the time this review was done (it was not clear that the drug caused the problem in all four cases; more recent evidence implicates just one case of liver inflammation). This extremely unusual side effect seems to result from a very rare autoimmune reaction

Do not take atomoxetine at the same time as a monoamine oxydase inhibitor (MAOI)—the combination can have potentially life-threatening adverse effects.

to the drug in which the body's immune system attacks and inflames the outer layers of the liver. To be safe, people with a history of liver damage or other liver problems may want to avoid using this drug.

✔ The package insert for atomoxetine warns of a possible increase in suicidal thinking from this drug, though not in suicide *attempts*. It's important to note that this risk was not found for teens or adults. Even for children it remains questionable because the methods by which the information was collected in the initial clinical trials weren't entirely sound and the problem was noted at only one of the 23 sites involved in the study.

✔ Atomoxetine can also increase your heart rate and blood pressure, though even less so than the stimulants.

The most common side effects of atomoxetine are:

✔ Nausea or vomiting

✔ Dry mouth

✔ Dizziness or light-headedness

✔ Drowsiness

✔ Constipation

✔ Sweating

✔ Decreased libido (sex drive) or erectile dysfunction

✔ Insomnia (far less common than with the stimulants)

✔ Irritability (rare; same as with the stimulants—some people actually report improvement in their mood or emotional self-control while on this medication)

 I couldn't handle the insomnia caused by the first stimulant I tried. My doctor tried me on other stimulants, and I had the same problems. But I'm not getting nearly as much improvement in my ADHD from Strattera. What else can I do?

This is a very unlikely situation, but it can certainly occur. Try some of the non-medication options in Steps Four and Five as well as ADHD coaching to see if any of these help. Some clinicians are combining atomoxetine with a stimulant while using lower doses of each in cases such as this. Discuss such combinations with your doctor if you think they might be beneficial for you.

The bottom line? Some studies suggest that atomoxetine may not produce quite as much improvement in ADHD symptoms as the stimulants. But you might find you get enough improvement to manage your symptoms and, at the same time, avoid uncomfortable side effects that can be associated with stimulants.

Atomoxetine might be a better choice than stimulants if . . .

- You have mild to moderate ADHD and don't need the most potent drugs, like amphetamine.

- You've tried stimulants without much improvement in your symptoms.

- You found stimulant side effects, notably insomnia, intolerable. Atomoxetine doesn't cause sleep problems.

- You or someone in your household has a history of substance abuse.

- You need the therapeutic effects all day long.

- You suffer from anxiety, depression, tics, nervous mannerisms, or obsessions and compulsions. Atomoxetine doesn't worsen these problems; in some cases, tics or anxiety might actually improve.

 Can I open the capsule to mix it with food or adjust my dose?

No. Atomoxetine has some acid-like properties that can burn the eye if you get some of the powder on your fingers and happen to rub your eyes. To adjust your dose, your doctor can combine various sizes of the capsules to better treat your ADHD.

Guanfacine XR (Intuniv)

This medication is based on a well-known drug used to manage high blood pressure in adults (guanfacine HCL), which now comes in a newer extended-release delivery system formulated for use in managing ADHD. To get the benefit of the extended-release system, you should swallow the tablet whole and not crushed.

The drug works reasonably well at managing ADHD symptoms in some patients but does not appear to be as effective as the stimulants (methylphenidate or amphetamine) and is perhaps slightly less effective than the nonstimulant atomoxetine. Unlike stimulants, which are eliminated from the body daily, guanfacine XR remains within the body for longer than 24 hours before being metabolized and eliminated.

The medicine works by an entirely different route in the brain than do the other ADHD medications. Those change the amount of neurotransmitter available in the brain at the synapse or gap between nerve cells, as discussed earlier. Guanfacine XR achieves its effects by fine-tuning the transmission of signals through nerve cells. Each nerve cell has small ports or openings (like sphincters or valves) along its main channel, or axon. These are called alpha-2 ports, and the more open they are, the more the nerve signals from that cell can be disrupted or weakened. Guanfacine XR closes these ports, strengthening signals as they move along the axon, which makes it easier for each cell to communicate with adjacent nerve cells, resulting in better functioning.

But because this drug is an antihypertensive, one of its side effects is a reduction in blood pressure that can lead to a subjective feeling of light-headedness and, in rare cases, fainting. Like other blood pressure medications, this one can cause drowsiness or sedation, and compared to a stimulant, it can take longer to adjust the dosage and find the right amount to get good control of ADHD symptoms.

The most common side effects of guanfacine XR are:

✓ Dizziness and drowsiness, especially when starting

✓ Headache

✓ Irritability

✓ Low blood pressure

✓ Nausea

✓ Stomachache

✓ Dry mouth

✓ Constipation

✓ Reduced appetite

✓ Very low blood pressure (uncommon)

✓ Slow heart rate (uncommon)

✓ Fainting (uncommon)

The side effects can lessen over time while the drug is being taken. Like atomoxetine, this drug has no significant effect on brain reward centers and thus has no significant abuse potential the way the stimulants might. It is often viewed as a third-line medicine for managing ADHD, given that it is less effective than the stimulants and greater patience is needed while adjusting the dose to achieve optimal results. Another drug similar to this type and FDA approved for children is clonidine XR. It may be approved for adults soon.

Bupropion (Wellbutrin)

• • • • • • • • • • • • • • •

Using a medication to treat a condition for which it is not FDA approved is called "off-label use" and can be perfectly safe (and even the best choice). But always ask your doctor to explain the pros and cons and why one drug is preferred over the alternatives.

• • • • • • • • • • • • • • •

Bupropion (brand name Wellbutrin) is a drug developed as an antidepressant that is sometimes used to treat adults with ADHD, particularly if they have associated anxiety or depression. It's not FDA approved for this use and hasn't been studied as thoroughly as atomoxetine for treating ADHD. But the research studies available do indicate significant benefits in managing the symptoms of ADHD, and the lack of FDA approval does not prevent doctors from prescribing it in cases where the medication might prove a better choice than either the stimulants or atomoxetine—generally when you have been diagnosed with anxiety or depression in addition to ADHD. Bupropion increases norepinephrine in the brain in the same way as atomoxetine, but it affects other brain chemicals too, such as dopamine, by which it may be benefiting ADHD management, and serotonin, which means it may produce different side effects than other approved ADHD medications that don't impact that chemical. If your only diagnosis is ADHD, you may be better off with either a stimulant or atomoxetine.

Other nonstimulants may be prescribed for you, but not necessarily for ADHD since none are particularly effective in improving ADHD symptoms. However, ADHD medications are often combined with drugs used to treat other conditions, such as antidepressants, antianxiety drugs, antihypertensive drugs, and even some mood stabilizer or antipsychotic drugs.

The antinarcoleptic drug modafinil (brand name Provigil) has shown some initial promise as a treatment for ADHD symptoms in children, but even these results have not always been replicated in other studies. There is also no research to date on use of the drug for adults with ADHD. The drug increases wakefulness and arousal and sometimes has been used to treat sleep apnea (disrupted breathing while asleep). But it has not received FDA approval for treatment of ADHD as of this writing because there was a rare case of a severe allergic skin reaction in the initial study submitted to the FDA as part of its approval process; the FDA has required that the drug be studied further for certain rare side effects before receiving approval. But the manufacturer, as of this writing, seems unlikely to invest any more time and money in this approval process.

15

What to Expect from Treatment

Medications for ADHD, especially the stimulants and atomoxetine, are among the safest, most effective, and best studied of all drugs used to treat psychiatric conditions. You have a very good chance—up to 80%—of zeroing in on a course of treatment that will turn your life around. It might take a little time. Some experimentation in consultation with your doctor may be needed to arrive at the best regimen for you. Here's how you and your doctor will get there:

A Physical Exam and Interview

You may have already covered these steps during your diagnostic evaluation. But if you were diagnosed a while back and are just considering medication now, your doctor will probably want to cover this ground again. It's wise to make sure no new factors that could affect a course of medication have entered the picture.

Your physician will conduct a physical examination with particular attention to:

✓ Your heart rate

✓ Your blood pressure

✓ Other medications you are taking

> Once you've started medication, immediately tell your doctor if you experience any significant heart functioning problems—palpitations, rapid heart rate, chest pain, dizziness, or fainting.

Rule out heart problems: If you read Chapters 13 and 14, you know it's important to identify any heart problems (either in yourself or in your family history) before deciding on a stimulant and probably even a nonstimulant. Some physicians may want to do an electrocardiogram (ECG). While not usually necessary, it's a fairly inexpensive precaution and not a bad idea if you haven't had one for any other reason in a long time.

Identify possible drug interactions: Although these drugs are safe in combination with most other medications, you want to ensure that you're not going to end up taking two stimulant medications at the same time or that you're not considering atomoxetine if you're taking an MAOI. If you smoke, discuss this with your doctor if he or she is planning on giving you a stimulant. Nicotine can also act as a stimulant, and the combination of the two can cause increased heart rate or blood pressure, or other stimulant side effects.

Finding Exactly the Right Medicine

• • • • • • • • • • •

Designing the best possible treatment plan is as much art as science. Try to be patient during the process: You're the one who has everything to gain!

• • • • • • • • • • •

You have about a 75% chance of responding to whatever ADHD drug is tried first. Don't be surprised if you feel like you're suddenly able to function pretty normally, maybe for the first time in your life. But if that doesn't happen, don't be discouraged. Lots of other medications, forms, and dosages are available for you to try and may still work for you. Overall, you have an 80–90% chance of responding positively to one of the various ADHD medications on the market in the United States at this time.

How will the doctor decide what to try first?

Stimulant or Nonstimulant?

This question is faced by every physician in every case of adult ADHD. Some start with a drug they've already been using successfully with a lot of their patients. Some start with whatever they were trained to use as a first-choice drug. Some use what their colleagues are already using extensively, especially if they have less experience than their colleagues.

Most doctors are likely to try a stimulant first if you don't seem to have another disorder besides ADHD, or it's urgent or a priority to get relatively rapid control over your ADHD (you are about to be fired if your work doesn't improve, your spouse or partner plans to leave you if things don't turn around quickly in your relationship, you're about to fail college classes, and so forth). The form chosen for a first trial might be determined by the pros and cons listed in Chapter 13. But my colleagues and I believe a doctor can home in on what's best for *you* by using more than standard guidelines. The checklist on page 147 will give you an idea of whether a stimulant or nonstimulant, like atomoxetine, might be best for you. You could also pass this list on to your doctor for consideration.

Yes	No	Issue to consider
☐	☐	1. Have you had an adverse or poor response to stimulants before?
☐	☐	2. Have you *never* had a prior adverse or poor response to a noradrenergic agent?
☐	☐	3. Is an immediate medication response *not* necessary for urgent management of your ADHD?
☐	☐	4. Do you have problems with anxiety or depression in addition to ADHD?
☐	☐	5. Do you have a tic disorder or Tourette syndrome?
☐	☐	6. Do you have significant insomnia or problems falling asleep?
☐	☐	7. Do you have significant problems with emotional impulsiveness, anger, or conflicts with others in the early morning?
☐	☐	8. Do you have any concern over using a Schedule II stimulant (possibly due to adverse publicity or abuse potential of the stimulants)?
☐	☐	9. Will you encounter conflict or hostility from family members if you take a stimulant?
☐	☐	10. Are your doctors or you concerned about the greater logistic difficulties of using a stimulant (frequent office visits, closer monitoring, and associated increased medical costs)?
☐	☐	11. Are you a college student for whom recreational misuse, theft, or diversion may be a potential problem?
☐	☐	12. Do you have a history of drug abuse?
☐	☐	13. Does anyone living with you, such as an immediate family member, have such a history?
☐	☐	14. Have you suffered significant insomnia from taking a stimulant in the past?
☐	☐	15. Have you experienced significant morning irritability, anger, or other behavioral problems while taking a stimulant?
☐	☐	16. Have you experienced blunting of affect or abnormal restriction of emotional expression (blandness) on a stimulant?
_____	_____	**Totals:** Total count of "yes" and "no" boxes checked

The more "yes" answers you give, the more I believe you should consider atomoxetine or another nonstimulant before going on a stimulant. Your doctor might also consider combining the two—using lower doses of each—to give you better (broader) coverage of your various concerns while limiting the occurrence of the typical side effects arising from each.

> If you think you're not benefiting from a drug you're trying, be sure to ask for feedback from someone who lives with you or is otherwise close to you. Sometimes the changes you're experiencing are easier for others to see.

Arriving at the Right Dosage

The dose it takes to treat ADHD successfully varies widely from person to person. Some adults require very small doses, equal to those used for children, while others need much higher doses, well above the average. Expect your physician to play with the range of doses for you, starting with a low dose and increasing it every week until you have a good response or such annoying side effects that going to an even higher dose is no longer an option.

But be patient. Sometimes it can take 2–3 weeks or even 1–2 months to find the best dose for your situation.

> The chances are quite good that the first medication you try will work for you:
> - You have only a 10–25% chance of not responding to the first drug tried.
> - You have only a 3–10% chance of not being able to tolerate the drug at all.

> Your doctor should always treat the most impairing or life-threatening condition first. If, for example, you have bipolar disorder or serious depression, the first medication tried should be for that condition, before you start an ADHD medication.

If the first drug tried does not work for you or work as well as you and your doctor would like, several other options may well be the right ones for you.

Let's say you try a methylphenidate delivery system such as the time-release pellets Ritalin LA or Focalin XR without much success. The delivery system, not the particular medication, might be the problem. Switching to the water-based osmotic pump Concerta or skin patch Daytrana might work for you. Failing that, switch to an amphetamine delivery system, like Adderall XR or Vyvanse, or to the nonstimulant atomoxetine

(Strattera). If these medications don't work for you, a trial on guanfacine XR might be indicated. A physician should go off label and use a non-FDA-approved drug for your ADHD only if you have shown no positive response to any of the others or you have another condition that needs to be treated first. In that case, bupropion might be an option for managing your ADHD.

Monitoring the Treatment

Medications designed to treat ADHD target the specific problems in the brain discussed in Step Two. Once you've landed on the right medication for you, you'll notice that:

✓ You're more productive at work

✓ You're better at sticking to tasks you need to do

✓ You can work better independently of others

✓ Your impulse control has improved

✓ You're more thoughtful about what you're doing

✓ You can better organize your thoughts

✓ It's easier to carry on conversations

✓ Your time management seems to be better

✓ You can now stick with boring tasks like writing business letters or reports without as much effort

✓ You're following through on promises

✓ Your emotions are under better control

At the start of your medication treatment, your doctor will probably want to see you or at least speak with you weekly to adjust the dosage as needed until your symptoms are controlled as much as possible. Afterward, you'll have to contact the doctor monthly if you're taking a stimulant, since most states require that you get a new prescription each month; refills are not allowed. Typically, this prescription must be filled within a few days to a week, and it can't be filled outside the state or the county in which it was written. Atomoxetine is not a controlled drug and can be refilled several times before a new prescription is required. The same is true for guanfacine XR.

Once you've found a dose that works for you, your doctor will likely need to see you for routine follow-up exams every 3–6 months. We've found that people often need additional dosage adjustments after the first 3–6 months on their medication, whenever they've had an unusual weight gain or loss, or when their life circumstances have changed dramatically and so has control of their symptoms. For instance, returning to college full-time could increase your need for time management, self-organization, and self-motivation skills, necessitating an increase in your dose, at least for the days you're in the classroom or studying. Or if you're a computer salesperson, you might find you need only small doses to manage your ADHD on days when you're calling on many customers in a region but more medication on days when you have stacks of paperwork to do, or should you get a promotion to district sales manager. Ordinarily, though, without such a marked change in circumstances or weight, once a dose has been established for a few months it typically can remain stable for many months afterward.

To help you monitor any changes in your symptoms, you might consider using the ADHD Symptom Tracking Scale at the end of this chapter. It can give your doctor more precise information about how medication may be improving your symptoms and whether additional dose increases might be necessary. It can also help you remember to pass on to your doctor far more specific information than you might recall without recording it.

When should the medication be discontinued? Doctors typically recommend that adults take their medication 7 days a week, year-round, because the impairments ADHD can produce occur not just at work or in college but in many other areas of life, such as driving, raising children, home responsibilities, managing money, and social relationships, all of which may benefit from medications for ADHD and might be affected detrimentally if the medication were stopped. So long as you're experiencing impairments in any of these areas, medication should continue.

Yet there may also be times when going off the medication might make sense, at least temporarily. In my clinical experience some adults have found that the medication they were taking greatly restricted their range of emotions and even creativity. While this is not common and has not been documented in research studies, these individuals were in unique employment situations where their complaints made some sense.

One such person was a poet. She took her medication most days because of the responsibilities she had running a household, paying bills, driving, and the like, but found that she was far less creative as a poet on the days that she set aside for writing. So, she would stop her medication for just those days, and the arrangement worked well for her. Poetry is nothing without its emotion, imagery, and metaphor, and she found her emotion was greatly restricted by her medication.

Another was a talented musician who played with a nearby symphony. Like the poet, he found that the medication was very useful for days when he was not playing his cello in the symphony and just doing routine household tasks, paying bills, or reading. But when he performed with the orchestra, he was much more connected to and expressive of the emotional tenor of his music—the qualities that had made him such a successful musician—if he went off his medication.

 Is the effectiveness of medication likely to be influenced by any major changes in the body, like a major weight gain or weight loss or hormonal changes (perimenopause/menopause)?

Some people, particularly growing children, do find that their dose must be adjusted with time. This is likely due to weight gain, growth in height, and other changes with maturation. These are less likely to be issues in adults, but some adults have reported changes in the effectiveness of their medication with weight changes. Therefore, doses may need to be adjusted from time to time, though less often than in children. We have no evidence about the impact of perimenopause or even monthly menstrual cycles on medication effectiveness, although they do worsen ADHD symptoms in some women, so this is a question that remains unanswered at this time.

It's Not Always about ADHD

Keep in mind that no medication for ADHD will miraculously solve all your problems. Troubles at work, in relationships, and elsewhere are not all caused by ADHD. Naturally, then, medication for ADHD won't erase them just because it is working. Unfortunately, figuring out which ongoing problems in your life need to be addressed by some other route can be tricky.

> Is your girlfriend always mad at you because you still forget to call her when you've promised to? Or because you two are just incompatible?

> Were you passed over for promotion because you don't know what to say and not say to your boss? Or because you haven't acquired the skills needed for the next job level?

> Are you being harassed by a collection agency because you don't pay your bills on time (or at all)? Or because you just don't have enough money for the debts you have taken on, or maybe they've just mixed you up with someone else?

In many cases, the first problem in each situation described may well be a consequence of having ADHD, while the second would not—and would not be expected to change as a result of taking an ADHD medication. Many people with ADHD find that it's easier to sort out the answers to these questions once medication is helping them think more clearly. For some it takes practice. Living with untreated ADHD for a long time can leave you with a history of mistakes you didn't need to make. Those mistakes can leave other people expecting bad behavior and poor decisions from you. In turn, you can end up resentful and defensive. Even now that you can function better, you might have trouble looking objectively at what's causing your problems. Do other people see what they expect based on your past rather than the way you are in the present? Has all the criticism you've received over the years left you expecting blame, seeing malicious intent where none exists? ADHD can leave you with a pile of unproductive attitudes and shoot-yourself-in-the-foot habits that are hard to shake. That's why many adults with ADHD recruit therapists, counselors, or life coaches to help them start fresh.

Giving Medication a Helping Hand

Therapists and life coaches can be of huge assistance to many adults with ADHD once they have begun a course of effective medication. Please understand, though, that there is no scientific evidence this kind of treatment will suffice on its own. It can, however, help you face the specific, unique issues you're dealing with. Or it may help fill in the gaps left when medication is simply not sufficient to address all aspects of your ADHD or at times of day when medications simply cannot be used.

The Resources at the back of the book list organizations and support groups that can help you acquire life skills, and sources for referral to therapists and life coaches.

Numerous strategies and tools for dealing with any remaining symptoms and impairments in the various arenas in which you operate are at your disposal. Consulting a psychologist or coach is one way to tap into them. Another is to read the rest of this book. Steps Four and Five offer a raft of techniques for improving your daily life. All of them are based on my theory that ADHD is a disorder of self-control, a condition that leaves you without a good sense of time. All are based on the principle that ADHD isn't a matter of not knowing what to do, but of not doing what you know when you need to do it. Add these methods to medication and you're well on your way to a better life.

ADHD Symptom Tracking Scale

Name: _____   Date: _____

INSTRUCTIONS FOR SECTION I

This form is designed to obtain your opinion on how often you demonstrate the following behavior. Please circle the number next to each item that describes how often that behavior has occurred during the period indicated below. Place a check mark (✓) by one of these time periods to indicate what period of time you are considering when completing this form. Then share this form with your doctor to give him or her more complete information about your usual level of ADHD before starting medication or during the initial phase when you begin taking medication.

_____ During the past 6 months (baseline)

_____ Since starting medication

_____ Since the medication dose was changed

_____ Since stopping medication

Symptoms	Never or rarely	Some-times	Often	Very often
1. Poor attention to details or careless in my work	0	1	2	3
2. Fidgety or squirm when seated	0	1	2	3
3. Can't sustain attention to tasks or leisure pursuits	0	1	2	3
4. Struggle to remain seated when expected to do so	0	1	2	3
5. Don't listen when others speak to me	0	1	2	3 (cont.)

Symptoms	Never or rarely	Some- times	Often	Very often
6. Restless	0	1	2	3
7. Have trouble completing instructions and so don't finish tasks	0	1	2	3
8. Find it hard to be quiet in leisure activities	0	1	2	3
9. Poorly organized in tasks	0	1	2	3
10. Feel like I need to be busy or "on the go"	0	1	2	3
11. Procrastinate work that requires prolonged effort	0	1	2	3
12. Talk too much	0	1	2	3
13. Misplace stuff I need for tasks or things I must get done	0	1	2	3
14. Blurt out answers before others finish what they are asking of me	0	1	2	3
15. Distractible	0	1	2	3
16. Can't wait for my turn at activities I do with others	0	1	2	3
17. Trouble remembering things in routine tasks	0	1	2	3
18. Interrupt what others may be doing	0	1	2	3

(cont.)

INSTRUCTIONS FOR SECTION II

To what extent do the problems you circled above interfere with your ability to function in each of these areas of life activities?

Activities	Never or rarely	Some-times	Often	Very often
In my home life with immediate family	0	1	2	3
In social relations with others	0	1	2	3
In my activities in the community	0	1	2	3
In school or other learning environments (if involved in an educational setting)	0	1	2	3
In sports, clubs, or other organizations	0	1	2	3
In driving	0	1	2	3
In leisure or recreational activities	0	1	2	3
In managing my money and finances	0	1	2	3
In my dating or marital relationships	0	1	2	3
In raising children	0	1	2	3
In my handling of daily chores or other responsibilities	0	1	2	3

Step Four

Change Your Life
Everyday Rules for Success

ADHD can make you feel like you're on a treadmill. Your symptoms make it much harder for you than for others to meet the demands of adult life. Some tasks don't get done by the deadline. Others elude you day after day no matter how hard you try. You can end up exhausted at the end of the day and still feel like you haven't gotten anywhere.

Fortunately, the medication that normalizes many people's symptoms can level the playing field. In fact, as I've said before, many of the adults I've known with ADHD declare that effective medication has completely turned their life around. If you feel that way after you've worked with your doctor to find the right medication, you might be tempted to close this book right now.

Feel free to do so. Put the book down and get on with the rest of your life.

Just keep the book where you can find it easily. I hope you'll come back to it soon, because taking Step Four can give you a valuable edge:

- *The principles you'll learn in Step Four augment your treatment,* kind of the way diet and exercise augment insulin for diabetes. Even with effective medication, you may experience some residual symptoms; the rules that follow can do the "cleanup."

- *The eight rules for everyday success provide you with backup for particularly hard times.* A major life crisis, physical illness, or any other stressful event might temporarily change the efficacy of your medication. Having an "emergency tool kit" on hand can keep you on a successful path at those times.

- *If for any reason your medication becomes less effective, the rules in Step Four can fill in while you and your doctor figure out a new medication regimen. Again, it's always wise to have a Plan B.*

- *The rules help you break old ingrained habits instilled by ADHD symptoms.* Even with medication helping you override the deficits of ADHD, old habits can cling. These rules remind you that there's a different way to conduct your daily affairs so you can get on with living a good life without delay.

Remember, in Chapter 11 I said there's a lot you can do to shape your environment so that it suits your needs. Step Four is all about learning certain underlying principles that will help you do that in your daily life. **Change the situation enough, and you reduce how handicapped or disabled you will be within it.**

. . . .
Disorders belong to people. Handicaps belong to situations.
. . . .

Each of the eight rules for success is based on the symptoms of ADHD and their roots in the brain. Follow them and you're directly counteracting the tendencies created by your ADHD brain that you read about in Step Two. Throughout Step Four I'll help you connect the dots between the greatest difficulties ADHD causes you (which you identified in Step Two) and the rules that will be most important for you to learn and follow. Use these rules whenever you want to succeed:

- When you need to get things done
- When it's important not to make mistakes
- When you need to be on time
- When you want to keep learning from the past so you can prepare for the future
- When you want to reach your goals so you can end your day knowing you may be tired, but at least you have something to show for it!

16

Rule 1: Stop the Action!

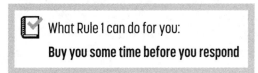

What Rule 1 can do for you:
Buy you some time before you respond

If you have adult ADHD, Rule 1 is for you. It's as simple as that.

The problems with self-control that are at the heart of ADHD begin with difficulty resisting impulses. Your boss proposes doubling your sales goals for the year, and before you can bite your tongue you bark out a laugh and say, "Are you *crazy?*" At the first sight of your neighbor's new lawn ornament you tell him it makes his house look like a cheap motel, and now he's not speaking to you— again. You see a gorgeous pair of designer shoes in a store window and rush in to buy them even though every penny of the paycheck you have in your purse is already spoken for.

By not stopping before you act, you allow no time for thinking. That thinking includes using your hindsight and foresight to get a feel for the situation, recall what has happened before, and consider what you should do next. It also includes giving yourself time to talk the situation over with yourself, using your mind's voice to consider how to deal with the situation.

Fortunately, you are not entirely without mental brake linings. But even with the full benefit of any medication you're taking, learning to stop reacting quickly to events around you with impulsive decisions, comments, and actions is going to take practice. Remember, the executive functions give you the capacity to exercise self-control. Making a conscious effort to use that capacity is up to you.

Start by getting a handle on *where* you are most likely to behave impulsively and where it can be most damaging

Go back to Chapters 6 and 7 to see what insights came to you about where and how your impulsivity has harmed you.

for you. There are times and places where it's OK to be impulsive, talkative, spontaneous, or capricious—or where it's at least unlikely to cost you much of anything (like a large party or raucous nightclub). But there are times and places you already know of where behaving this way can cost you dearly (work, college, intimate relationships).

Figure Out Where Impulsivity Hurts You Most

Don't just guess at the answer. If you need to, compile a list of these costly situations from your past experience. Ask your spouse, your partner, a good friend, or a sibling to help you pinpoint your trouble spots. Write them down or ask the other person to do it for you so you have a reminder of where to be on guard and where to practice "stopping the action" most.

Where is impulsivity a big problem for you?

At work?

Where and when?

_____

_____

While dating?

What typically happens?

_____

_____

In conversation?

With whom—a friend, partner, spouse, or other loved one?

_____

_____

When you shop with a credit card?

What stores (or websites) and items do you find irresistible?

_____

_____

When you get behind the wheel of your car?

    Always or only on certain routes or at certain times?

_____

_____

Other?

_____

_____

Strategy: *Perform a simple action to stave off the urge to act.*

Before you enter one of the situations you just identified, the next time the occasion arises, I want you to practice buying yourself a few seconds to give your thinking a chance to kick in by *performing any of the following simple actions:*

✓ Inhale slowly, exhale slowly, put on a thoughtful expression, and say to yourself, "Well, let me think about that."

✓ Just say, "Hmmmm, let me see now" pensively after inhaling and exhaling.

✓ Put your hand over your mouth for a few seconds.

✓ Or just put your hand on your chin as if in a thoughtful posture as a cue to keep your mouth shut and not say the first thing that comes to mind.

Almost any small action will do. In Chapter 9 I mentioned an adult who mentally locks his mouth with an invisible key to prevent himself from speaking. Once you've ingrained the habit of using public, outward actions to buy yourself time, you can shift to using mental gestures like that. For now, try a more public version of the locking trick: Put your hand behind your back or in a pocket and perform a key-turning motion.

To buy even a few more seconds, paraphrase what the other person just said to you:

✓ "Oh, so you want to know about. . . . "

✓ "You're asking me to. . . . "

✓ "What you need done is. . . . "

✓ "You feel that. . . . "

Again, these are just examples. Pick a phrase that's easy for you to remember, that will roll off your tongue easily, so you're likely to use it.

The key is not to say or do anything else in those first few seconds. Notice I did not say don't do *anything*. You've undoubtedly been told to stop and think many times before, but no one ever tells you how you're supposed to curb an incredibly strong urge to act or speak and just stand there and do nothing when every molecule in your body is urging you to do something. The reason this little ploy works is that it does give you something to do while you're buying the time to think that ADHD usually denies you.

Practice: Try to practice doing this often, every day, lots of times a day, even when you're alone. This behavior comes naturally to those without ADHD because the motor system of their brain is not as quick to fire off as yours is. It may be unconscious for them, but it has to be very, very conscious for you—at least at first. The more you practice, the sooner it will become an unconscious habit. It will be hard, but believe me, it's worth it! You are going to try doing this so often that people may look at you funny: Why does this guy always have his hand on his chin or over his mouth? Why does this woman constantly repeat back to me what I've just said? Try not to worry about it; it's better than getting an angry, shocked, or disgusted reaction. If you're having trouble developing a thick skin about others' responses to you, check out Rule 8.

Strategy: *Pick a slow-talking model and play that role when you converse.*

You gotta stop playing Tigger and become Winnie the Pooh. Quit being a Robin Williams in some rapid-fire stand-up comedy act and start being more thoughtful, like Tom Hanks or Will Rogers. Slow it down. Think of yourself as a southerner instead of a northerner. Even just taking a little extra time to utter a sentence will give that theater in your mind time to load up the DVD of your past experience and get the camera playing on your mental screen. Practice speaking slowly in the mirror. See yourself as your slow-talking role model. Speaking more slowly will give your frontal lobes a chance to get some traction, to get engaged instead of being swept along in the incessant tide of your impulses.

Following Rule 1 helps you buy time to let your private mental home theater gear up and show you some video of your past experiences that may pertain to the present situation. Having bought that time, you must now consciously try to think about the situation. Thinking here means visualizing your past relevant experiences to find out what they have to tell you. The next rule will help you do this.

17

Rule 2: See the Past . . .
and Then the Future

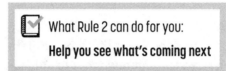

> What Rule 2 can do for you:
> **Help you see what's coming next**

When a problem arises during your day, are you often completely thrown about what's likely to happen and what to do? Do you constantly beat yourself up for making the same mistakes again and again? Rule 2 is for you.

You already know that your mind's eye (nonverbal working memory) is not as powerful as those of people without ADHD. This makes it really challenging to activate your mental imagery related to hindsight and foresight before taking action. You may very well already look back at your life and even look ahead for what your experience can tell you is going to happen, *but only after you've already acted and the dust has settled.* The good news here is that being able to exercise hindsight at all tells you that you do possess the capacity. The bad news is that exercising hindsight only after the fact usually leads directly to beating yourself up for having done or said the wrong thing. On top of the criticism of others, self-blame can beat you right into the ground, and you might find it harder and harder to get back up.

> Go back to Chapter 9 to remind yourself of the specific difficulties with the mind's eye that sounded familiar when you read the "Nonverbal Working Memory" section.

As to foresight, being able to extract from past experience what's likely to happen in the future is great—as long as you can do it on the spot in the situations where you need that forecast. A decision you made last week to do something differently is likely to evaporate before you have a chance to follow through.

You need a way to make sure that what you learned from the past stays accessible when you need it.

Identify Where You Have Weaknesses in Nonverbal Working Memory

Figure out where you have the most trouble looking ahead; those are the places where you'll most want to practice seeing the past.

Do you hit every problem with a "hammer," because they all look like "nails" to you?

Adults with ADHD haven't compiled a large store of remembered past experiences, so the subtle differences among problems and the need for different tools to solve them often elude them.

Does learning anything new require you to go through a long, slow trial-and-error process?

If you can't call up mental images easily, you have to keep trying one thing after another.

Do you have trouble saving money, sticking to a diet, or perfecting an athletic skill?

Deferring gratification is tough when you can't keep calling up the mental image of the prize that lies ahead.

Strategy: *Use an imaginary visual device to turn on your mind's eye.*

Learning to stop the action gives you that mental space to turn on the mind's eye. But your mind's eye is so fragile that the next irrelevant thing that happens around you can fracture what you were trying to think about. Suddenly your mind is off, wandering to whatever tangent that distraction suggested to you. So what you need to do is mentally call up some visual device that you usually find engrossing. Your big flat-screen TV? Your favorite video or computer game? The minicam on your smartphone? Right after you stop the action, click on this device. You can even use a surreptitious physical motion to turn it on right when you're saying "Hmmmm" or right after you've used the same hand to make a locking motion.

Now try to focus your mind and literally see for yourself, on the screen of that device, whatever light your past may shed on this particular situation. Visualize what happened the last time you were in a situation like this. Get creative. See the past unfolding in all its colorful, detailed action, as if you're filming it or replaying it right in the space that you're in.

Practice: The more often you do this, the more habitual and automatic it will become, and the more different "videos" will pop into your mind from your memory bank to guide your future. You'll be able to think: "Wow, the last time I interrupted a meeting with a joke, everyone laughed at *me,* not the punch line." Or "I felt really guilty when I got home with those shoes and discovered my son needed some expensive books for school and I didn't have the money." Don't just practice projecting the mind's eye onto a TV or computer monitor in your highest-risk situations. To cement the habit, do it where it's easiest to do—where the stakes are lower, there's no pressure, and it's easier for you to stop the action and give yourself the opportunity.

Strategy: *Use tangible visual aids to give your mind's eye extra help.*

More on this in Rule 4. But let's say there's a particular setting where your mind's eye is blind and you're tired of beating yourself up for not seeing what you should have done. Shoot a photo, clip one out of a magazine, or draw a picture of something that represents the "don't." Do the same for one that represents the "do." Put them up where you can see them often, reinforcing those mental circuits that connect what you want with what you've done in the past that has put it out of your reach. The woman whose downfall was expensive shoes posted inside her closet door a designer shoe ad coupled with a photocopy of her bank statement showing a zero balance. Opposite that she posted a picture of her son and a photo she clipped from a magazine of a high school diploma. Seeing it every day helped the same images pop into her head when she passed by her favorite shoe store.

Your mind's eye (nonverbal working memory) may be weaker and less effective than that of others. But you also have a mind's voice. And that can serve to enhance what you are trying to visualize in your mind. Read on to Rule 3.

18

Rule 3: Say the Past . . . and Then the Future

 What Rule 3 can do for you:

Help you analyze the situation before deciding what to do

Help you develop rules you can use for the same situations in the future

Do you see what's coming and still go with the knee-jerk response? Do you feel like you keep having to learn the same lessons over and over? Rule 3 is for you.

Nonverbal working memory—the mind's eye—isn't enough for most of us if we want to operate successfully in the adult world. Not only do we need to see what happened the last time we took a certain course of action. We also need to be able to analyze each situation before us and weigh the pros and cons of different responses. Let's say you know that blurting out your opinion in the middle of the last meeting was a mistake. When your boss presents a new plan that you think is misguided at this week's meeting, do you just clam up? Write your thoughts in a memo to him later? Recruit some allies and tell him about your misgivings together? Come up with an alternative plan?

We need to be able to distill rules and guidelines from what we experience so that we get better and better at responding and planning as time goes on. Waiting till after an open meeting to express an opinion that might not be received well is one example of a rule you could adopt in the workplace. Knowing who your allies are among coworkers might be a good guideline for getting ahead in your job and career.

The key ingredient in these mental processes is *language*. When we learn to stop the action and then see the past so we can foresee the future, the only way to learn from the mental imagery is to use words to describe it. Talking to ourselves is central to problem solving. It's essential to planning. It's even critical to understanding the rules of society. Weak verbal working memory, in fact, is why it's not uncommon for adults with ADHD to rack up a criminal record, often of misdemeanors. It's not malevolence that causes the lawbreaking but a fundamental failure to apply or follow the rules at key moments in life, usually because of impulsiveness. Unless you talk to yourself about your options, it can be pretty easy to decide, for example, that shoplifting something that's caught your eye is OK because you are not likely to be seen or you can always return it later.

Having a grasp of what ADHD does to your executive functions can really help you compensate for deficits. Yes, your mind's voice (verbal working memory) is weaker and less effective than those of people who don't have ADHD. On the other hand, if you practice using it and make it stronger, you can use your improved verbal working memory to compensate for a weak *non*verbal working memory. And vice versa. Talk to yourself about the mental images you're able to call up and you strengthen those visual memories for later use. Enrich your bank of visual memories and you have more information to analyze logically with your mind's voice. The bottom line? You improve the odds of your making better, more nuanced decisions.

Identify Your Biggest Verbal Working Memory Problem Areas

What did you learn about your mind's voice in Chapter 9?

Developing verbal working memory skills is a relatively sophisticated achievement. To start practicing, try to come up with a modest goal you haven't been able to reach due to poor verbal working memory. For example, you may really want to manage your own investments, but it might make sense to start with a simple savings plan that requires you to deposit a small amount of cash in a savings account every week first. Even a simple-sounding goal is a lot harder to pursue consistently than you might think before you start.

Strategy: *Become your own interviewer.*

Don't just see the mental images in your mind:

✓ Discuss them with yourself.

✓ Label them.

✓ Describe just what you are seeing in your mind's eye.

✓ Then extract some rule or principle from this review that tells you what you want to do the next time you face this situation.

That voice in your head is not just there to keep you company. It's a device to help with self-control.

Literally picture yourself holding a microphone and interviewing yourself on TV. Verbally describe the situation you're in. Ask yourself relevant questions. Be as tough on yourself as the most dogged journalist. Ask yourself questions like these:

✓ "What's going on here?"

✓ "Have I been in a situation like this before?"

✓ "What's the same and what's different?"

Do you have trouble reading other people's emotions?

With particular people and in particular situations or all the time?

_____

_____

Do you find it very difficult to understand and follow rules?

Where and when?

_____

_____

Do you have trouble understanding and retaining what you've read?

_____

Do you decide to begin a diet, a savings plan, or another program and then drop it almost immediately?

_____

✓ "What did I do last time?"

✓ "Is that an option here?"

✓ "Are there better choices?"

✓ "If I decide to do X, what will happen?

✓ "Have I seen X [a successful person you admire] do this? If not, what has X done in similar situations?"

✓ "If my decision turns out badly, how will I feel tomorrow?"

Strategy: *Narrate what's happening out loud.*

As you know, kids narrate their own play all the time. As adults, we're supposed to have learned how to make this commentary private and internal. Unfortunately, ADHD has other ideas. So let's go back to what worked so well when we were kids. Go ahead and describe what's happening to you in all the rich, vivid language you can come up with *out loud*. You don't have to make it *loud*; just *out* loud. Externally vocalized words, even when just whispered, are more powerful at controlling and guiding our behavior than words we may say in our mind. You might feel most comfortable doing this when you're alone. You certainly won't want to do it where you could disturb someone. But it's possible to choose situations where you can practice this without fear of someone else's reaction:

> **Even if you're around other people, you can pretend you're using a hands-free device, talking on your cell phone. You'll blend right in with everyone else.**

✓ When you're working on a project at home and trying to decide whether to keep at it or abandon it for something more fun

✓ When you're trying to stick to the rules of the road while behind the wheel and you're alone in the car

✓ On a jog or walk through the woods when you're planning what you're going to do with the rest of your day

Just take the solitude as an opportunity to get used to verbalizing where you are, what you're doing, what you could do next, and what might happen. While you're at a task, give yourself instructions about keeping at it, doing it carefully, completing each step, and finishing the project. You'll find you're much more likely to see the task through to the end than if you just thought about these ideas in your head.

Your mind's eye and mind's voice aren't as strong as those of other people. You can give them a boost by following Rules 1–3. But there's even more you can do to help yourself: see Rule 4.

19

Rule 4: Externalize Key Information

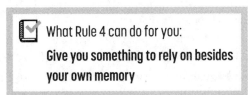

✓ What Rule 4 can do for you:
**Give you something to rely on besides
your own memory**

**Are you forgetful and scattered? Do people treat you as if you're unreliable and
untrustworthy? Are you beginning to agree that you have no self-discipline or
stick-to-itiveness? If you have adult ADHD, you probably answered yes to all
of these questions. Rule 4 is most definitely for you.**

Even with ADHD robbing you of some of the power of your executive functions, you can build them to their greatest potential. That's why it makes such
sense to follow Rules 1–3. The more you practice the strategies in the last three
chapters, the more you build those skills despite an innate deficit. That doesn't
mean you have to stop there, however. You deserve all the help you can get in
leveling that playing field.

I can't emphasize enough how important it is to avail yourself of the many
ways you can boost your internal memory with external cues. Kids with ADHD
get this kind of help in school when the teacher provides periodic reminders to
stay on task. Parents set up star charts to motivate children to keep up the efforts
they're making with chores or homework. Parents also often use picture charts
that graphically break down the steps in routines like getting dressed for school so
that a child who gets lost or distracted in the middle of the process has something
to consult to stay on track.

Can you think of any reason why you shouldn't get the same kind of assistance?

The difference for you, of course, is that you're generally on your own here.

You might be able to enlist the aid of a spouse or a roommate to some extent, but for the most part it's up to you to create and use external reminders. The good news is that it can be fun. You get to use the abundant creativity bestowed on many people, including those with ADHD.

Where Do You Still Have a Lot of Trouble . . . No Matter How Much Mental Effort You Invest?

Some of the tools you can include in your arsenal are listed in Chapter 10.

It doesn't really matter whether your difficulty is with stopping the action, seeing the past, or saying the past. The strategies for externalizing information can be applied to any type of reminder you need. You can—and should—use external cues all the time. Many of the tools that are perfect for issuing reminders are imminently portable and adaptable, meaning there's no limit to how and where you can take advantage of them. Still, it will help to know which areas seem to be particularly memory resistant for you so you can be sure to tackle them and spare yourself the frustration of ongoing shortfalls.

Do you still have lots of trouble staying silent when it would be better to do so?

When and where?

_____

_____

_____

Do you forget to gather tools or materials for the tasks you need to do?

At work or elsewhere?

_____

_____

_____

Does your mental to-do list always include items that get carried over from day to day, never getting checked off?

Which kinds of tasks?

_____

_____

_____

Do you feel like you're often at the mercy of your emotions?

Which emotions are a particular problem for you (such as anger, frustration, guilt, shame)?

_____

_____

_____

Do you have less control in some situations or with certain people than others?

_____

_____

_____

These are just a few problems that can be solved with the help of externalized information. Think of the "blunders" or "failures" you regret the most—that's where you can immediately apply one of the following strategies.

Strategy: *Put physical cues in plain view in problem situations.*

These cues can take many forms. Here are some examples keyed to particular problem situations:

✓ A sign you put on the margin of your computer monitor or on your desk within your visual field reminding you not to start surfing the web instead of doing your work. Or try a picture of your boss on which you have printed "Get to Work!" Or, do as Homer Simpson did in one memorable episode when he displayed a picture of his young daughter, Lisa, with the statement "Do it for her!" beneath it.

✓ A note to yourself that you keep in the same pocket as your wallet so that when you reach in to pull out the wallet and buy something you get the note too—and it asks you whether you really need to make that purchase. Better yet, make it a sticky note taped right onto that credit card.

✓ A card you tape on your smartphone screen that asks whether that call you're about to make can wait till later, after you've finished whatever task you're in the middle of doing.

Your physical cue must be in plain sight, right in the place where you need the reminder.

✓ A photo of the tennis trophy (or any prize) you want to earn to keep you practicing.

✓ A symbol, like a stop sign, that you can put anywhere to remind you to stop the action before making any decision.

✓ A list of rules for writing a complicated report that you have to generate every 2 weeks at work.

An external cue not only helps you stop what you were impulsively about to do but also tells you what to do instead, and even why you were trying to change yourself for the better in the first place.

Physical cues are your stand-in for a shaky working memory. Something external, in front of us, is a far more potent reminder than an image or word held in our mind. Next time you enter the situation for which you've created a cue, your cue will catch your attention and remind you of what you intended to do in that situation.

For example, do you impulsively eat too much and want to lose weight? Put a picture of the latest hot athlete, or film star, or your own younger, slimmer self on your refrigerator. You could also post a stop sign on the refrigerator door that says, "Step away from the refrigerator," perhaps accompanied by a picture of a police officer you found in a newspaper or magazine and clipped out to tape alongside your stop sign.

Strategy: *Make a list of steps or procedures you want to follow the next time you encounter a problem task.*

To-do lists are used by everyone, ADHD or no ADHD, *because they work so well.* If you end your day dejected because too many of the goals you set for the day fall by the wayside, a to-do list can be a godsend. If you put it where you can't miss it, it will remind you of what you need to be doing right now, or next, when you drift away toward something more fun or just something that entered your field of vision and was hard to ignore. There's nothing like the feeling of checking off that last chore or task at the end of the day. *Now* you can have some fun!

> *I tried to use to-do lists, but I guess I got just as carried away writing the list as I do with other things that I get immersed in. I didn't know when to stop and had a three-page list of things to do in a single day. I just couldn't seem to see when I wrote it that I was being insanely unrealistic about how much I could get done in a day. How can I rein myself in and write a reasonable to-do list?*

One idea, if you have a sympathetic spouse, a mentor at work, or a sibling or roommate who's willing to pitch in occasionally, is to ask someone else to review your list. Remember, one of your biggest stumbling blocks is a poor sense of time. This can make it really tough to figure out how long each item on your list should take (to say nothing of how to budget your time while you're working on that list!). Many adults who don't have ADHD have a pretty good idea of how long standard household tasks usually take. A mentor or boss at work will know how long work jobs take. And you can start to develop a sense of how much longer than the average person you might need to do particular tasks, depending on your skills in that area, how interesting you find the task, what the distractions usually are, and what your attention span is usually like.

Which brings me to a second idea for reining in an out-of-control to-do list: use a journal. If you keep track of how long you took to do certain tasks, you'll begin to know yourself and your habits well enough to budget your time more accurately. See the following strategy.

Strategy: *Carry a journal with you all the time.*

A journal can help you record the specifics of certain tasks and what it takes you to get them done, as just noted. But more generally it can serve as your record of what you need to do. One of the greatest difficulties you're likely to have with working memory is remembering what others have told you that's important. How often have you disappointed yourself or someone else by forgetting:

✓ A date?

✓ A commitment?

✓ A promise?

✓ An appointment?

✓ A deadline?

Whether at work, in social relationships, or at home with your family, the ability to remember what you've said you'd do is crucial to your integrity and your image in the eyes of others. This is especially so for promises you make to others. As I'm sure you know, for you it's more routine to forget this sort of information than to remember it. I'm sure you also know how dearly you pay for these lapses—at work, at home, and elsewhere. The adults I know with ADHD report that being viewed as more forgetful and less reliable than other adults—being unable to keep and fulfill promises and commitments the way adults are expected to do and generally being thought of as less trustworthy—causes them more shame and distress than just about any other shortcoming that ADHD has handed them.

If you carry a purse, putting your journal in an outer flap where you can see and reach it easily is much better than putting it inside the zipped or snapped main compartment, where having to fumble for it might deter you from entering important information.

You don't have to resign yourself to that fate. Start carrying a journal with you, as already noted in Chapter 10. This can be a small blank notebook, a bound journal, or anything else you can write in, including the electronic devices mentioned in Chapter 10. The point is you have to take this with you all the time.

Just as you put your wallet in your back pocket or purse, you should have a small paper journal or a smartphone for note taking on you at all times!

Today, before you have a chance to forget, start using your journal: Write in it anything someone says to you that you are to do, any promise you make, any commitment to others, date, deadline, meeting, or other time-sensitive instructions—*anything and everything that may be important for you to remember.*

Don't consider yourself completely dressed in the morning until you slip that journal and pencil or other note-taking device into your pocket.

Smartphones or digital recording devices are ever present and may seem like an obvious choice for your journal. *But I've found that people are likely to use and remember to read a small pocket journal, whereas they often misplace their little digital recorder or just forget to replay and listen to what they said earlier.*

Don't just write in your journal. Refer to it often, hourly if need be, to keep yourself on target in honoring your agreements, completing assigned work, fulfilling promises to others, and meeting those deadlines. Set your smartphone alarm to ring every 15 to 30 minutes to remind you to check that journal. If you are an adult with ADHD, this journal should be with you at all times unless a situation calls for you to be naked. Even then, it should be right nearby, within easy reach, if you have to remember anything during this time.

A journal is invaluable: It's your external working memory.

As I said, adults with ADHD report that it's awfully depressing to be viewed as unreliable and immature. It doesn't take long to agree with others' assessment and view yourself as devoid of persistence, self-discipline, and willpower. To help address your executive function deficit, follow the next few rules.

20

Rule 5: Feel the Future

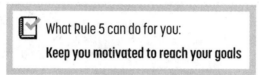

> ☑ What Rule 5 can do for you:
>
> **Keep you motivated to reach your goals**

If the purpose of the tasks you need to complete feels flat and abstract to you, leaving you uninspired to keep at them, Rule 5 is for you.

One major consequence of what I call the *time blindness* of ADHD is difficulty conjuring up the past so you can apply what you recall to the future. That's why Rules 2 and 3 are so important: They help you learn from your memories so that you become more adept at handling similar situations up ahead. But ADHD also leaves you with large gaps between the *present* and the future: If no one is dangling a carrot right in front of your face, you may need lots of convincing to keep moving toward your destination.

Sometimes the self-talk you learned in Rule 3 will keep you going. Telling yourself that you *need* to get this job done, telling yourself *how* to do it, reminding yourself of the *steps* you need to take along the way, and nudging yourself to pay attention to the *time* can work in many situations. Another method that might keep you at a task is to warn yourself about what will happen if you *don't* do what you're supposed to do. This form of "saying the past" might involve reminding yourself that you had to pay a lot more for your son's textbook when you weren't able to buy it early because you had spent the money elsewhere. It might mean listing the jobs you've lost because you didn't meet assigned deadlines. It could be telling yourself that your husband didn't speak to you for a week after you made an excuse to leave his father's birthday party early because you were bored.

Unfortunately, for adults (and kids) with ADHD, the threat of negative consequences isn't the most potent incentive. And even if it were, not everything comes with an obvious, direct, or dire consequence for nonperformance. For many adult goals, you're just supposed to do what you have to do because it has to get done and getting it done is the right thing to do. A lot of adults in the general population find this intrinsic motivator pretty unmotivating too. Many people who don't have ADHD turn to the same types of incentives described in this book, at least for some tasks they really don't want to do. **With ADHD thrown into the mix, however, those incentives become essential.** Here's why:

✓ ADHD can make it tough for you to grasp the moral imperative behind getting a task done for its own sake, so that's not likely to move you.

✓ ADHD can turn uninteresting into agonizingly boring, making you feel like you're going to explode with restlessness if you can't get away from a task that's no fun.

✓ ADHD can make it impossible to see that what you do may have not just one bad consequence but two or three, each of which can lead to its own six knock-on undesired outcomes, and that each of those can produce twelve others, and so forth.

✓ And a poor sense of time can prevent you from grasping that all these consequences can unfold much faster than you'd imagine, before you have a chance to jump in and stop the avalanche.

Figure Out Where You Are Least Motivated to Get Things Done

In which area do you find it hardest to stay motivated?

School? _____

Work? _____

Household chores? _____

Community activities? _____

Relationships? (Which ones?)

_____

_____

What items grow old on your to-do list because you don't feel motivated to finish them?

_____

_____

ADHD makes it hard to stay motivated to complete tasks for all the reasons listed above. But there's another reason that various responsibilities seem so uncompelling, their purpose so flat and abstract: **There is no emotion attached to getting them done.** Emotion is an extremely powerful motivator. In fact, our emotions are the very source of our self-motivation.

> Scientists studying human emotions have concluded that a major function of emotion is to cause or motivate us to act. Although emotions are complex, certain emotions generally lead to certain types of actions. Here are just a few examples:
>
> - Fear leads to "fight or flight"—attacking the source of danger or running away.
>
> - Anger leads us to right a wrong.
>
> - Joy and pleasure lead to the urge to keep doing what we're doing.
>
> - Shame dissuades us from repeating the shameful act.

Even our self-talk often relies more on emotion than we realize. Consider again how we warn ourselves of the negative consequences of not finishing a task: It's not just the practical aspects of those consequences that we find undesirable. Sure, having to spend more money than necessary on a textbook hurts your bank account. Losing jobs hurts your bank account too. And receiving the silent treatment from your spouse disrupts your daily routine. But what may really move us to heed the warnings we give ourselves is our memory of how we *felt* about these consequences. Leaving your son without a textbook he needs until you can come up with the cash might make you feel shame. Being fired repeatedly is pretty humiliating and devastating to your self-esteem. And being shunned by the person you love most really hurts and might make you angry too.

· · · · ·
Visualize it →
Verbalize it →
Feel it
· · · · ·

For some people, the memory of these uncomfortable feelings is enough to motivate them to do what they need to do to avoid a repeat performance. That's why you need to use *your visual imaging of these past events and their emotions to help you trigger the motivation you may need to get things done.*

Recalling or anticipating the negative consequences of not doing something is not as powerful a motivator for most people as focusing on the potential positive consequences of getting it done. Focusing on the negative can even get you down compared to the uplifting, rejuvenating, and inspiring feelings you can get by imagining how great it will feel to get to your goal.

> **Strategy:** *Ask yourself point blank, "What will it feel like when I get this done?"*

After seeing and saying the past to foresee the future, your next step is making a conscious effort to really feel what it will be like when you finish the task at hand or reach your goal. Ask yourself, "What will it feel like when I get this done?" and then focus on that emotional sensation. What could it be?

✓ Pride?

✓ Self-satisfaction?

✓ The happiness you anticipate from completing that project?

✓ The sense of accomplishment you may experience?

✓ The pleasure or happiness of others with whom you have shared this goal or for whom you are doing this job?

Whatever that emotion is, work hard to feel it, right then, right there, as you contemplate your goals. Then keep doing this throughout your work or as you pursue this goal or project. Every day, or every time you are in that situation, working toward that goal or destination, repeatedly ramp up your efforts to really feel what it will be like when you get there.

All future-directed behavior needs a motive, and all motives (motivations) are the consequence of our emotions. Your imagined emotions, brought forth with a lot of conscious effort, can be the fuel that drives your activities, boosting you toward your destination like a cruise missile. People without ADHD also propel themselves forward by imagining what reaching a desired destination will feel like. The difference is that they can usually do it without much thinking or effort because their sense of time and their visual working memory are strong enough to allow such foresight easily. For you, however, this has to be a very conscious, deliberate effort.

> **Feel that future, and keep feeling it, all the way, until you get there!**

Give this technique a boost by cutting out pictures of the rewards you hope to earn from what you are doing and placing these around you while you're are working. They'll enhance the potency of your own imagery and therefore make the emotions you're anticipating even more vivid.

So, work on visualizing, verbalizing, and then feeling not just the goal and the steps you need to achieve it, but also what you will feel when it finally gets done. Every time you sit down to continue working on a project, task, or goal, one of the things you must do is to *feel* that future outcome.

In Chapter 9 I suggested that calling up mental images of past accomplishments can relieve stress and anxiety when you're under the gun, leaving you feeling both calm and motivated. If you have trouble imagining how you'll feel when you get a job done, start by recalling a similar task that you *did* get done. This is a perfect example of how each method you use to thwart an executive function deficit caused by ADHD boosts your ability to use another compensating strategy. So this is another reason to practice following Rule 2: The more mental images of past successes you've collected, the easier it will be to imagine the positive feelings you'll have when you complete the task before you right now.

A good reason to practice Rule 5 is that it will fill up your inner emotional well. The same time blindness that keeps you from having as large a mental store of visual or verbal memories as those without ADHD also causes you to have fewer palpable, vibrant, potent, or motivating emotional memories. It's not that you don't feel the emotions that others feel. It's just that you may not have your experiences with them slotted away in your mind to the same extent. Or they may not be as easily retrievable as they are for people who aren't dealing with ADHD.

This strategy, like those under the other rules in Step Four, makes it easier for you to accomplish what you want right now, in this moment. But the more you practice it, the more memories and skills you build, making it increasingly easy in the future. So, "begin with the end in mind," as Stephen Covey says in his bestselling book *The 7 Habits of Highly Effective People.* Visualizing the goal and feeling that sense of accomplishment, relief, pride, and success you will have, not to mention seeing the rewards you may earn, can help to fill up that motivational fuel tank you need to get through the work you have to do.

Meanwhile, though, you have more strategies at your disposal; turn to Rule 6.

21

Rule 6: Break It Down . . . and Make It Matter

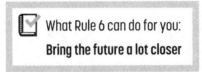

What Rule 6 can do for you:
Bring the future a lot closer

If pictures, words, and feelings are too fleeting to keep you on track, Rule 6 is for you. Actually, we've found that virtually everyone with ADHD benefits from following Rule 6. Difficulties sustaining attention and seeing past the present make it awfully hard to conjure up all the motivation you need internally. You need a little help from the outside. Fortunately, the possibilities for getting it are numerous and fairly easy to access. It's all a matter of bringing that oh-so-distant horizon into closer focus. But first, see if you can get a sense of why the future always seems so far away:

What Makes Your Destinations Seem So Distant?

ADHD can make the future seem hopelessly distant. A goal that requires a significant investment of time, incorporates waiting periods, or has to be done in a sequence of steps can prove so elusive that you feel overwhelmed. When that happens, many adults with ADHD yield to the temptation to find an escape route. Maybe you literally run away, going AWOL at work or calling in sick. Maybe you shift your focus from figuring out how to get the work done to figuring out how to shunt the responsibility to someone else. Maybe you've learned to act the class clown. Or you might have crafted other smoke screens to obscure the truth that you've made no progress and have no idea how to start inching forward. Feeling helpless makes some adults with ADHD regress to relying on a willing helper to cover for them by picking up the slack. Of course, none of these tactics helps you get done what you need to get done. And none of them protects you forever from others finding out that you haven't fulfilled your obligations. Better to figure out where you're stymied most and use external motivators appropriate for those situations.

Do you panic or simply go blank when someone gives you a deadline so distant you can't even imagine that far ahead?
  Where does this typically happen in your life?

_____

_____

Do complex projects overwhelm you?
  What types do you usually have to tackle?

_____

_____

Do you have a lot of trouble working without supervision or camaraderie?
  Where and when?

_____

_____

These are just a few simple questions to get you thinking about when you feel blocked from moving forward on a project or goal. Reading about the following strategies you can use to provide yourself with external motivation may bring up more examples.

Strategy: *Break down longer-term tasks or goals into much, much smaller units or work quotas.*

It's so easy to lose sight of the end point of a project. If even an end-of-the-day deadline seems remote to you, you'll want to use this strategy for most work goals and some household goals. If you have a big project—like cleaning out all the closets in your house or preparing next year's budget for your department at work—this strategy will be even more crucial. And you'll need to break the project down even further. In fact, the longer a project will take to complete, the more steps it's likely to involve. The further the deadline, the more essential it is to break it down and the smaller you need to make the chunks of work or other actions required.

✓ *If a project has to be done before the end of the day, break it into 1-hour or, better yet, half-hour chunks of work.* Write down what you need to get done in each period of time and then run a highlighter over the step you're working on right now to keep your attention focused on that and off the rest of the units.

✓ *If you have a project that has to be done by the end of the week, first figure out how much you need to get done each day.* With something like closet cleaning, this can be as straightforward as assigning one day for each closet. If it's something more complex, where the tasks depend on each other, you may have to work a little harder to figure out the appropriate sequence of steps. If you're at work, ask your boss or mentor to help you. Use other people's reports of the same work from the past; the office files, electronic or paper, should help. Talk to friendly colleagues who have had to complete similar projects and see if their breakdown could work for you.

Then look at the goal for each day and break it down into 1-hour or half-hour segments. Or if, as is often true at work, you need to intersperse this project with others, pick a time period to dedicate to this project, write it into your day planner or the calendar on your desk, and then when the time comes break that period into even smaller time segments during which you will complete each of the steps for a certain task.

A classic example of this occurred during the 2016 Summer Olympics when Michael Phelps, an adult with ADHD, was showcased on TV and the commentators were giving a lot of background about him. They showed his daily schedule, which was broken into 15-minute units from the time he arose early in the morning until bedtime. It contained not just his planned training workouts for that day, but even how much time he would give himself to eat meals, nap, and devote to his favorite leisure activities.

You don't necessarily have to plan your day to this degree, but it would help to plan your time at work just like Michael did to help keep yourself focused on your goals and work assignments. So, mark your day planner beforehand with how you plan to spend each hour of that workday. Then break that hour into 15-minute units, assigning each a microtask you hope to do that is part of the bigger project in that unit. Doing this helps collapse what might seem like an endlessly long project into a series of quick-moving bites of time and accomplishment.

✓ *Keep in mind that the breaks between these chunks of time are just as important as the productive periods.* Don't be embarrassed to think of yourself in the same way you'd think of a young student with ADHD: You wouldn't expect a child to come home from school and do 30 math problems in one sitting (nor would a good teacher expect that in the classroom). You ask the child to try just five. When those five are done, you let the child with ADHD take a break for a minute or two. Then you give him just five more. Five at a time is not overwhelming, even for someone with ADHD, but 30 can be. Just do five at a time and do that six times in a row with short breaks in between, and you've got your 30 problems done. I know several professional athletes with ADHD who use this tactic while doing their workouts or weightlifting. Instead of saying they will bench-press a certain weight 30 times, they specify 10, then say, "That was easy" and immediately do 10 more, and so on. We all take "baby steps" toward any difficult goal. Why should you be any different?

> **Sign to post on your desk or work area: CHUNK IT, BABY!**

Strategy: *Make yourself accountable to someone else.*

This strategy doubles your external motivators. Not only are you breaking down a complex or extended project into smaller tasks, but now you're bringing another person into the mix, someone who will know whether you're doing what you set out to do. We are far, far more likely to follow through on the goals we set for ourselves if we tell someone else what we're doing and how we plan to do it (by chunking it, usually) and then notify that person when we achieve each smaller objective. Most of us care a great deal about what others think of us, and this social judgment of others adds even more motivational fuel to our inner fires to get things done.

> **Making yourself accountable brings in the internal motivator of emotions too. Letting someone else down doesn't feel good; receiving admiration feels great.**

> **Make yourself accountable to someone for reaching each small subgoal and also the final project goal.**

✓ At work, make yourself accountable to a supportive coworker, supervisor, or mentor.

✓ At home, use a supportive partner, spouse, roommate, or neighbor.

Reward your helper. In the final strategy of Rule 6, you'll learn how important it is to reward yourself as an incentive to keep working toward your goals. Well, this goes for the person you're asking to help you stay on track too. Thank and reward this person so he or she doesn't feel burdened by this process. A helper who feels appreciated by you is likely to take satisfaction in helping you achieve your goals. That person is also likely to want to keep being your coach and mentor.

Strategy: *Give yourself little rewards as you accomplish each small objective.*

When we design programs for children with ADHD, we invariably give them points, tokens, poker chips, or some other reward for achieving the small work quotas discussed above. This, along with praise and approval, helps them get and stay motivated to finish drawn-out work assignments. The same applies to adults, except there is no teacher to dispense the points or rewards. You have to do that for yourself.

We all do this. While writing this chapter, I told myself that if I wrote for 30 to 60 minutes and got five pages done, I would make myself a cappuccino in our nearby kitchen. Then if I did another five pages or more, I could pick up my bass guitar, which I keep in my office, and practice (yet one more time) a sixties rock tune I am trying to master, but just for a few minutes, one time through the song. If I wrote five more pages, I could have a Hershey's Kiss off the nearby coffee table or a can

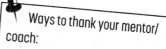

Ways to thank your mentor/coach:

- Take him out to lunch every couple weeks
- Bring a token gift periodically
- Offer a small gift certificate to a store she likes
- Bring him his favorite coffee or tea in the morning or soda in the afternoon

of Diet Coke from my office fridge. Or I could just take a minute to appreciate the beautiful view from my second-floor office window across a tidal creek and marsh behind my home.

Use whatever turns you on; the lesson here is the same: Give yourself brief little rewards for getting your small quotas done and then, brick by brick, you will be amazed at just how much work gets done across the longer term. That's how I wrote this entire book—brick by brick. Or, as Anne Lamott put it in her book on writing, *Bird by Bird*: Her brother had to write a class paper on birds and could not get started, so their father told him to just write a few sentences on one bird, then come tell him about it, and so on, until the paper was finished. So, my friend, take it bird by bird. Stop briefly to note your success and briefly reward it at the end of each bird.

What small rewards could you easily give yourself?

At work: _____

At home: _____

Elsewhere: _____

Putting it all together: OK, so you have broken your work into smaller quotas, chunking it all the way. Just as important as using smaller quotas to get bigger ones accomplished is what you do once each chunk or quota is done. Do at least these four things:

1. Congratulate yourself.

2. Take a short break (a few minutes).

3. If someone is available, tell him or her what you've gotten done.

4. Give yourself a reward or a taste of some privilege or activity you enjoy but make it small and brief.

All three of these strategies are going to help motivate you to get things done that you have not previously been able to finish or to get to those longer-term life goals you really want to attain but never seem to get started on or complete. All are ways to artificially motivate yourself. When visualizing, describing, and feeling the emotions associated with completing a task are not enough to sustain your focus . . .

✓ Chunk it.

✓ Make the goal and smaller quotas public.

✓ Take brief breaks.

✓ Reward yourself after each one.

Rule 7 will give you more ideas for making the external world boost your internal motivation.

22

Rule 7: Make Problems External, Physical, and Manual

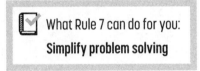

What Rule 7 can do for you:
Simplify problem solving

If you typically get lost in all the possibilities when you try to mentally solve a problem, Rule 7 is for you. Because your verbal and nonverbal working memory capacities are weakened by ADHD, you probably find it challenging to hold all the relevant facts in your mind when presented with a problem to be solved. Weighing the pros and cons, listing the tools or materials you need, analyzing the merits of various approaches, figuring out risk/benefit ratios—all of these operations are difficult to carry out strictly in your head. It's not that you're incapable of logical analysis or you lack intelligence—far from it. It's just that you need to make the process tangible and external to move through it smoothly and successfully. In essence, you need to be able to use your senses to oil the gears of your mind:

✓ You need visual aids so you can scan all the facts and questions in front of you.

✓ You need to be able to physically manipulate the information to make it real and manageable.

✓ You need to make the problem external so that trying to solve it doesn't rely so much on your working memory—and so your emotions don't erupt with the frustration of trying to do it all in your head.

Know Where the Most Complicated or Urgent Problems Come Up in Your Life

This is a tricky assessment to make. What's hardest for you, the abstract problems that come up at work or the emotion-laden issues you have to deal with at home? Solving problems for yourself or solving them for others? Having to think on your feet or having to systematically work through complicated options? Knowing where you're most paralyzed by problems will help you develop the external aids most likely to make your life easier.

How successfully do you solve problems at work?

Which ones are toughest for you—budgeting, coworker relationships, teamwork, dealing with supervisors, other issues?

_____

_____

How successfully do you solve problems at home?

With your spouse/partner? _____

With your kids? _____

With siblings? _____

With parents? _____

How successfully do you solve problems in your social life?

In dating? _____

With friends? _____

With neighbors and in community groups? _____

How successfully do you solve practical problems?

Repair needs (such as home or car)? _____

Shopping (such as dealing with store employees)? _____

With vendors (such as utility companies, credit card companies)? _____

Know What Kinds of External Aids Help You Most

Most people have some sense of where their perceptual strengths are. For those with ADHD, who need to rely comparatively more on their senses to assist their thinking, it's important to know:

What type of learner do you think you are?

    Visual (you need to see the material laid out before you to grasp it)? _____

    Auditory (you need to hear it to have it make the most sense)? _____

    Tactile (you need to touch it to get a full sense of it)? _____

    Kinesthetic (you learn best by moving around in a physical activity)? _____

Do you remember what it was like for you to try to solve problems in your head when you were a child? Even the easiest mental arithmetic problems may have been impossible for you to do. If so, you probably also remember how demoralizing it was to be denied the use of beads or other tokens because conventional educational wisdom said that by your age you should have been able to do without them.

Our studies have shown that difficulty solving problems in their head keeps affecting people with ADHD as they get older, though in different ways. Young children may have trouble with mental arithmetic. They may not be able to recite backwards a string of digits read aloud to them. As they get older, they can't hold all the parts of a story in mind (characters, places, dates, actions, and the like) as well as other adults when asked to explain the story concisely or write a paper analyzing the story in some way. Our research now shows that this problem affects adults with ADHD just as much.

Lots of people with ADHD have bad memories of experiences like that. Fortunately, you're an adult now, and no one can tell you what tools you're allowed to use to solve the problems that come your way. You have dozens at your disposal. If they help you figure out where to spend your paycheck, how to talk your boss into a raise when company funds are tight, how to get a term paper done on time, how to keep the kids from bickering, or which home improvement project to tackle first, it's your *obligation* to use them.

We're all supposed to develop verbal and nonverbal working memory during childhood so that we can retain and call up mental images and so we can put words to what we've experienced. Later in our development we should be able to take those mental representations apart, manipulate them, move them around, and recombine them in various ways. Doing so is critical to:

✓ Coming up with various options

✓ Solving problems

✓ Inventing various ways of doing or explaining things

✓ Generally developing plans for the future

Unfortunately, the problems ADHD causes in the brain rob us of the typical development of these executive functions. So how can you compensate? Try this:

Strategy: *Use physical, external tools to solve problems whenever you can.*

Holding lots of information in your mind and manipulating it in various ways without losing track of anything is a pretty sophisticated ability. It also requires a fair amount of effort, energy, and concentration. Ask any adult who is trying to figure out how to squeeze a little more income out of the same old paycheck to fund braces or a new car at the same time as refereeing a fight between the kids and trying to get dinner on the table—all after a 10-hour workday. Exhaustion has a way of making mental problem solving almost impossible. I know many adults who take advantage of their computer to make lists or use sticky notes or magnets they can move around on a board, audiotapes, graphic devices, and other tools to get the data out of their already-cluttered minds and put it somewhere else where they can see it, feel it, hear it, or manipulate it. They use whatever it takes to give themselves a fresh take on the problem at hand.

You can do the same. After all, you probably have the same demands on your problem-solving abilities *plus* the interference of ADHD to deal with. Take all the help you can get.

Once you have all the data pertinent to your problem in pieces—on paper, using objects, or graphically represented in some other way—you can move all that physically represented stuff around with your hands, your eyes, your ears, even your whole body to see if a solution reveals itself. If it's a verbal problem, use paper, 3″ × 5″ file cards, or even a laptop computer.

Think of this as the "advanced" version of Rule 2. Rule 2 advised you to externalize something you need to remember by writing it down, posting it on a sign, or creating some other cue. Here in Rule 7 you extend the idea a bit further, externalizing everything you need to consider to solve a problem. Doing this can be as simple as doodling on a piece of scratch paper or sketching various parts of the problem as you think of them. There are lots of ways to make problems we're trying to solve physical in some way. Decorators make miniature two-dimensional furnishings and work with various room arrangements on a plastic form board in the shape of the room, house, or office. You can now buy computer software programs that let you do the same thing. Engineers and architects use simulators on computers all the time in designing roads, bridges, cars, or new chemicals and solving physical problems of all sorts. Landscapers do the same sort of thing with miniature props or computerized simulation programs. Carpenters, plumbers, tile and brick layers, and people in other trades manually manipulate pieces of the problem to be solved to get the job done. After all, isn't that what blueprints are for besides just instructing us in building something? We can tinker with the design on the blueprint better than in our minds.

For example, one adult with ADHD I knew was building a house. He knew that the kitchen was critical and needed to be designed properly as he and his partner would be likely to use it. So he took old moving boxes and literally built a mockup of their kitchen and its counters with these boxes. Then he walked through it, pretending to do things like cook, unload groceries, get to the fridge, and load the dishwasher. This allowed him to make critical readjustments to their initial floor plan to better accommodate the ways in which they use their kitchen.

If you have ADHD, odds are you will be better at solving various problems or completing various mental tasks if you can get them outside of you, broken down into pieces or in some other physical form that you can work with manually in addition to mentally. Try it. And if those around you raise their eyebrows as they see you "playing" with these "toys," invoke Rule 8.

23

Rule 8: Have a Sense of Humor!

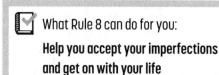

What Rule 8 can do for you:

Help you accept your imperfections and get on with your life

If you're still having trouble owning your ADHD, Rule 8 is for you. There's nothing like a little self-deprecating humor to help all of us accept our imperfections, get over any self-consciousness about them, and get on with the business—and pleasure—of living.

• • • • • • •

ADHD may be serious, but you don't always have to be.

• • • • • • •

All the preceding chapters of this book are a testament to just how serious a problem ADHD can be. You just know you are going to make mistakes, probably far more than most people. Having ADHD is certainly not your fault. So what can you do about it? Besides everything you've learned so far, try this:

Strategy: *Learn to say, with a smile, "Well, there goes my ADHD talking [or acting up] again. Sorry about that. My mistake. Now I have to try to do something about that next time."*

When you say this, you've done four very important things in a social situation:

✓ You owned the mistake.

✓ You explained how it may have happened.

✓ You apologized and made no excuses by blaming others.

✓ You promised to try to do better next time.

Amazing what you can do with a few short phrases. Do those things and you will keep your self-esteem and your friends and loved ones. Disown your ADHD conduct, blame others, find excuses, and make no effort at trying to be better and you will be social toast.

As we said in Step Two, know your ADHD, own it, and then work with it. You have to do these things if you stand any chance of mastering your ADHD. So don't deny your imperfections. Know them, own them, admit to them easily, and work with and laugh at them daily. That takes time to do. But then they become no big deal—and they won't likely be so again.

I still remind friends of 42 years whom I trained with as an intern in psychology—and they certainly still remind me—of the hound's-tooth black and white leisure suit I wore to a clinic one day at our medical school while training as an intern. And we all still laugh until we get tears in our eyes about what came to be known as a "full Cleveland" because I accented the outfit with a white belt and white shoes.

My ex-wife will tell you repeatedly with little encouragement of how I once did a cartwheel into a large hot tub at a spa resort in front of numerous attractive young ladies as I tried to enter the pool without using the railing or stairs. So much for graceful coordination. And just don't ask her about all the stop signs I have nearly run or actually missed due to my color blindness when those signs were in front of green bushes. And what of all the public speaking, newspaper photos, professional videos, TV programs, and other public displays I have been involved in that show my ever more balding and graying head, facial wrinkles, and those gold crowns that twinkle in the photo from the camera flash when I am caught smiling? I own every last one of these imperfections and then some. So? I like who I am, warts and all, I want to be a part of life, I have goals yet to achieve, and I intend to live this life as fully as time and opportunity permit, nonetheless. So should you. As one adult with ADHD told me, "I want to go sliding into my grave and know that I lived a meaningful life rather than slouch toward my final ending."

We want you to take much the same attitude toward your ADHD: You have it, so you might as well own up to it. And, whenever appropriate, laugh about it. It may be appropriate to laugh at yourself apologetically with others. It's almost always appropriate to have a private laugh at yourself. If you make ADHD a serious, all-encompassing disability, it will be, and that's the way others will treat it—and probably not want to spend much time with you. If you approach it with a sense of humor, they will too, and you can laugh with them about it (and about their imperfections too!). They'll probably end up wanting to spend more time with you as a friend.

Most important, though, you'll be able to live with yourself—with all your imperfections and all your struggles to deal with a condition that's not easy to live with. Treatment won't cure it or even address all of it, and therefore ADHD is most likely going to be with you for the rest of your life. So get used to it and smile about it once in a while. As great examples find Dani Donovan's artwork about ADHD and the videos of Jessica McCabe and Rick Green about the humor in ADHD, both available on the Internet, including Rick's original video, *ADHD and Loving It,* about ADHD and marriage.

To help you remember these eight everyday rules, photocopy this page and tape these rules to your bathroom mirror. I did this for years with Stephen Covey's *7 Habits of Highly Effective People.* I got to see and relearn them every morning. I know many others who did the same until they had memorized and could easily recite those fantastic principles for leading a productive, effective, and purposeful life of integrity. So, put these eight rules where you can see them every day, even keeping a second copy on your desk at work, another in your day planner, another taped beside your computer monitor, and copies in other places you are bound to be looking at repeatedly each day.

- -

Rule 1: Stop the Action!
Buy some time before you respond.

Rule 2: See the Past . . . and Then the Future
See what's coming.

Rule 3: Say the Past . . . and Then the Future
Analyze before deciding; develop rules for the future.

Rule 4: Externalize Key Information
Rely on something besides your memory.

Rule 5: Feel the Future
Stay motivated.

Rule 6: Break It Down . . . and Make It Matter
Bring the future a lot closer.

Rule 7: Make Problems External, Physical, and Manual
Simplify problem solving.

Rule 8: Have a Sense of Humor!
Accept your imperfections and get on with your life.

- -

Step Five

Change
Your Situation

Mastering ADHD in Specific Areas of Your Life

Take a quick look at the bar chart on the next page. It shows that adults with ADHD reported being impaired in every area of life, much more than adults without ADHD. These findings are probably no surprise to you. Self-control and a sense of time are critical to everything you do, everywhere you go. When they are hampered by ADHD, you feel it in every aspect of your daily existence.

Some activities and situations may be harder for you than others. If so, you might want to start Step Five by reading the chapters on the domains where you have the greatest ADHD-related difficulties. Or skim the chapters to see what they have to offer. You'll find a wealth of practical ideas for handling the specific demands of specific settings, all flowing from the rules in Step Four and all targeting the unique deficits associated with ADHD.

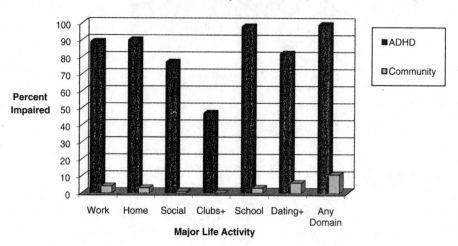

From *ADHD in Adults: What the Science Says* by Russell A. Barkley, Kevin R. Murphy, and Mariel-len Fischer. Copyright © 2008 The Guilford Press. Reprinted by permission.

24

Education

"My teachers in school were always telling me to read the directions on my school assignments carefully so I would know exactly what I was supposed to do. But, oh no, not me. I would always just lunge right into the work, figuring that I had a pretty clear idea of what I was to do. And so I would get a lot of my assignments wrong. I just could not seem to slow down and take the time to read the directions. I just wanted to get the work over with as fast as possible."

"I initially failed out of college for not doing my coursework. So I worked for 3 years, and then I returned to a community college and got my associate's degree. I finally transferred back to my original university, gaining acceptance back into the engineering school, from which I hope to graduate this year. But even that is not guaranteed, because I still have these unfinished papers to turn in for classes that already ended."

There's probably nothing harder for people with ADHD than getting an education. That goes for both children and adults. ADHD impairs academic performance, it leads to behavior problems in school, and it reduces the number of years of education completed successfully.

I may be giving you information you've already gathered firsthand. If so, you probably also know already that lack of a good education has a lot of downstream or knock-on effects. It lowers your earning potential, both annually and across your lifetime. It limits your choice of occupation. It can influence the kinds of friends you may have and the social circles in which you participate. It can leave you with low self-esteem, which can further hamper your social life.

Now that you're on track toward changing your destiny, you may find that you want to go back to school. If you don't have a high school diploma or a college degree, perhaps you've decided to get a GED and/or enroll in college. With the help you get from medication, you may feel confident that you could complete a training program, seminar, workshop, adult education program, or continuing education course to give your career a boost. Or maybe you're a young adult and still in the midst of your higher education. On the following pages I'll share a lot of practical tips for being as successful as you can possibly be, whatever your educational goals may be.

But first, you might benefit from having some idea of what you're up against so that you're prepared to seek any accommodations or assistance you might need. Why devote time and energy to education without giving yourself the best possible chance to succeed?

Know What You're Up Against

You can enhance your educational achievements through a number of routes, from medication to accommodations provided by the school to self-help strategies. Your best bet for targeting the aids tailored to meet your unique needs is to know as much as you can about your own abilities.

Have You Had ADHD Since Childhood?

If so, you've been struggling in school from the start. My colleagues and I have found that adults with ADHD who were diagnosed as children tend to have done worse in school than those diagnosed as adults. Why? It's hard to say for certain, but here are some possibilities:

✓ Some people who have gone through childhood without a diagnosis or treatment may have milder ADHD than those diagnosed at an early age.

✓ Those who managed without treatment may have had superlative individual support from parents and teachers.

✓ In some cases, high intelligence can compensate for ADHD symptoms in school just enough to make the adults in a child's life think a diagnosis is unnecessary.

For these reasons a child might remain undiagnosed and might be more successful in school than diagnosed children whose problems were so apparent that they led to early referral and diagnosis. When those bright children grow up, they often end up seeking help for ADHD. By adulthood parental support is no longer available to the same extent. And, as you read in Step One, the symptoms affect domains of life where intelligence can't overcome impairments, so the adult gets tired of trying to manage life with untreated ADHD symptoms.

So, if you were diagnosed as a child, you're probably facing more obstacles than if you were diagnosed recently. If your ADHD was relatively severe, you're dealing with greater deficits to begin with. On top of that, problems in school tend to build on each other over time. Both your performance and your self-confidence may have dropped over the years. It's important to know that so you can seek the degree of assistance you need to achieve your educational goals.

In recent research, my colleagues and I found the following in studies examining the educational history of both people diagnosed as adults and people diagnosed as children. The information on those diagnosed as adults came from the reports of people who knew them well as kids, mainly their parents. The information on those diagnosed as children came from a study I did with Mariellen Fischer, PhD, that followed children with ADHD in Wisconsin into adulthood (average age 27 years), at which time they still had the disorder.

School outcome	Adults with ADHD (%)	Children with ADHD as adults (%)
Graduated from high school	88	62
Graduated from college	30	9
Retained in grade	25	47
Received special education	35	65
Received other assistance	48	42

Do You Have Learning Disabilities?

A substantial minority of adults with ADHD also have specific learning disabilities (LDs). An LD is a delay in a specific area of basic academic skills, such as reading, spelling, math, and reading comprehension. You read in Step Two that the executive function deficits of ADHD can cause reading comprehension problems. But these problems are more striking in some people than others. If you score below the 14th percentile on standardized tests, you might be said to have a specific LD.

We know from research that these LDs are more common in adults with ADHD than in the general population. We've found particular problems in not just reading comprehension but also listening comprehension. Whether you qualified for a specific LD or fell just below that cutoff line, it's not hard to see how challenging learning would be if you couldn't grasp or retain what you'd read or heard in the classroom as well as your peers! An LD could also have a negative impact on your social life if others didn't realize you were having trouble understanding what they were saying and misinterpreted your reaction as lack of interest in them. Fortunately, even if any LDs you may have were not addressed when you were a child, you can get targeted help for them today.

The same studies cited above showed that adults diagnosed with ADHD as children had more learning disabilities than adults diagnosed as adults:

School outcome	Adults with ADHD (%)	Children with ADHD as adults (%)
Diagnosed learning disorder	28	45

Lay the Groundwork for Learning

The vast majority of adults with ADHD have experienced problems in their educational history. Besides the figures quoted above, our studies showed that adults with ADHD were more likely to have been punished at school (42% among those just diagnosed—a whopping 62% among those diagnosed as kids). They had more problems with others at school (44% and 53%, respectively). A huge 71% of adults diagnosed as children had been suspended or expelled at least once. Obviously, you're not looking to repeat that kind of experience. Yet you're likely to have problems again if you're pursuing adult education classes or workplace educational programs. You can do yourself a big favor by knowing what you can do to get around those problems.

You're Entitled to Reasonable Accommodations

If you're still in college, you'll probably need certain accommodations to help you succeed. And you should have them. You are entitled to reasonable adjustments to your educational activities as provided under the Americans with Disabilities Act. You may want to become familiar with the requirements for documenting your ADHD for your college if you wish to take advantage of these reasonable accommodations.

See the Resources for books that explain your protections under the Americans with Disabilities Act, the documentation you'll have to provide, and the types of accommodations that might be available.

Please keep in mind, though, that this law exists to help you help yourself. No accommodations can do the hard work of learning for you. Assert your right to accommodations, but don't stop there. Always be prepared to do whatever you can for yourself. You'll do much better in school if you do, and what you learn from helping yourself will transfer to every other setting you function in, from work to home.

Learn the Eight Everyday Rules for Success

Following the rules laid out in Step Four is one big way to help yourself. In educational settings, these rules should be your bible.

Medication

In all honesty, experience and much research tell us that self-help recommendations like these rules are often not enough by themselves to master the adverse effects of your ADHD at school. If you've been coasting along without medication but are considering going back to school or starting a challenging job, now is the time to reconsider this treatment. ADHD medications are the most effective way to begin to address the school and workplace problems that ADHD poses for most adults.

You'll probably find the long-acting ADHD medications most useful since they can manage your symptoms for 8–14 hours with only one or two doses a day. You may benefit from supplementing a single dose of the long-acting medications with a second dose of an immediate-release pill late in the day or in the early evening.

See Step Three for details on medications.

Find a Coach or Mentor

More on accountability in Chapter 21.

This is someone to whom you can make yourself accountable every day for the work that you believe needs to get done that day. This can be a teacher, professor, roommate, classmate, more senior student, or someone in the special student services office. If possible, meet with your coach twice a day for 5 minutes. Use the first meeting, usually in the morning, to review your to-do list or goals for that day. Then meet again late in the day to show your coach what you've accomplished on that list.

Identify the College ADHD Liaison

This person, who usually works in the special student services office, can do the following for you:

✓ Review your documentation that you have ADHD

✓ Describe the types of curriculum adjustments and other accommodations typically provided to students with ADHD so you can identify the ones you might need

✓ Work with your professors to see that you get them

✓ Link you up with psychologists, counselors, and physicians (usually psychiatrists) who work at the student counseling center

Get Tools That Can Keep You on Track before You Begin

✓ Use a *daily assignment calendar* to set goals for each day and track appointments. You'll use this calendar to review the day's tasks with your coach and also keep it in a visible spot to remind you to stay focused on your goals and appointments.

✓ Use your *journal* to write down everything you need to do, including assignments, individual requests made of you by teachers, meetings you've scheduled, promises you've made or that others have made to you—anything of the slightest importance. Review this journal several times a day to make sure you're doing the things you have recorded there.

> See Chapter 19 for tips on making the most of your journal.

✓ Get a *notebook organizing system* and *day planners* and use a *personal time management or organizing app* too if it will help you stay organized. (But be aware that smartphones and other such devices can also be incredibly distracting and markedly reduce your productivity due to text messaging, e-mail, or just surfing the Internet for fun. Think twice about using them—they don't always help distractible people.)

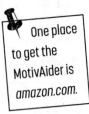

> One place to get the MotivAider is *amazon.com.*

✓ Buy *separate, colored folders* for each class, where you can keep your completed assignments. It's not unusual for adults with ADHD to do assignments and then misplace them and not be able to turn them in on time.

✓ Get a *tactile cueing device* that can provide frequent prompts to keep you focused on the work at hand. One possibility is the MotivAider, a small plastic box about the size of your cell phone that holds a small vibrator and a digital clock that can either be set for any interval you wish or set to random intervals so that it vibrates unpredictably.

Tips for Success

Scheduling Smart

✓ Schedule harder classes/meetings/work in your "peak performance" time slot each day. For most people, this may be midmorning or early afternoon, but people vary in the time of day when they're most alert. Some research shows that adults with ADHD find afternoons or even evening hours their best time to focus and concentrate, which is a few hours later than for adults in the general population. In any case, know your daily cycle of arousal and alertness and use that knowledge to schedule those tasks that require more concentration and effort into the best time slot.

✓ Alternate required or harder courses with elective or fun classes during the day or across the weekly schedule of your classes. You don't want to stack up all the hard classes on a single day or during the first few days of the week as this can overtax you, make you too tired to do well in them, cause you to lose interest or motivation partway through them, and ruin your attitude toward school. Interspersing the hard stuff with classes or activities you find more interesting or entertaining, or just exercise workouts, ensures that you're never faced with too many classes or projects that demand lots of effort too close together. You can do this at work as well by arranging your work so that you alternate difficult/demanding with easy/interesting tasks on a given day.

Getting the Most Out of Classes

For information on the Smartpen, which records as you take notes, see livescribe.com.

✓ Tape or digitally record important lectures or meetings or use the Smartpen digital recorder.

✓ Get any extra curriculum materials your teachers may have available or have set aside at the library especially for their classes, such as videos that supplement what you're learning in class and additional notes or articles that further explain the topics that are being covered.

✓ Some adults with ADHD in college settings have been able to get assistance with note taking in class if their writing problems are particularly severe.

✓ One way to stay awake, alert, and focused is to do something more active while you have to pay attention. If you have to write down the gist of what is being said in a lecture, you are more likely to stay attentive than if you just sit and observe. Take notes continuously, keeping your hand moving, even if you don't really need to write down the information.

✔ Exercise before exams or boring classes. Routine aerobic exercise makes a person able to concentrate for 45–60 minutes longer than usual directly afterward. Learn to build in brief exercise breaks throughout your day, especially before you have to do something that you find difficult to concentrate on. Just 3–5 minutes of exercise may be enough to help you concentrate better. If the class is long enough that you're being given beverage or restroom breaks, use them to do some quick aerobic exercise, even if it's just faster than normal walking outside the building or in the hallway.

✔ Use small-muscle exercises while engaged in boring classes or studying. Repeatedly squeeze a tennis or stress ball, tap your feet while studying, chew on some gum or even a rubber toy of some kind, or pace while you read. Any movement seems to be helpful to adults with ADHD when they need to concentrate on some task.

Handling Homework

✔ Use your computer rather than writing out papers and other assignments by hand. People with ADHD often have motor coordination or other handwriting problems that make handwriting slower and less legible. In college, you may also be able to tape or digitally record some of your assignments and turn in the recording as your report if you have a history of significant writing problems. The special student services counselor mentioned above can get you this type of curriculum adjustment with your teachers if you require it.

✔ If you have lots of reading to do for school or work, learn to use the SQ4R method for reading comprehension. Here, briefly, is how it works:

- Survey the material to be read—just leaf through it quickly to get some idea of how much is to be read, how it is broken up, and so forth.

- Draft some questions that need to be answered from what you are to read. Often these are at the end of the chapter to be read or have been given to you by your teacher.

- Now use the **4R**s: **R**ead just one paragraph, **r**ecite out loud in a soft voice or whisper what was important in that material, **w**rite that material down in your notebook, then **r**eview what you just wrote.

- Do this for each paragraph. This not only makes you review what you're reading four times per paragraph (read, recite, write, review) but also gives you frequent mental breaks as you shift your concentration at the end of each paragraph from reading to reciting to writing to reviewing across the assignment. As you get good at this, you can read longer passages, such as two paragraphs at a time or an entire page, before engaging in the recite, write, and review steps. This is a great strategy for people with working memory problems.

Passing the Test

✓ Should you request extra time on timed tests? Many young adults with ADHD in college settings believe or have heard from others that this may be a useful accommodation to request. But what little research there is on the subject is not that clear. Everyone, disabled or not, seems to benefit from extra time to take timed tests, but that does not mean it will necessarily help compensate for your ADHD or solve your problem with taking these tests. More recent opinion suggests that you're better off using a method called "time off the clock." This involves using a stopwatch to take these timed tests. With this stopwatch you will not get any more time to take the test than do other students, say 1 or 2 hours. But what you are allowed to do is to stop the watch anytime you like, as often as you like, to take a short break of a minute or two. Use this to stand up, stretch, walk about the room or into the hallway, get a drink of water, use the bathroom; then return to your test and start the stopwatch. When you've used up all the test time on the stopwatch, you're done. Yes, this will result in your taking more time than others to complete the test, but that is just a by-product of the real accommodation here, which is self-pacing the exam. You're not given more active work or face time with the exam than anyone else. The strategy that you're using is the point here: breaking up the test into smaller work quotas and having frequent self-determined breaks to briefly refresh your mental focus and concentration.

✓ Take timed tests in test settings that are free of distractions or offer greatly reduced chances of being distracted.

An Extra Boost

✓ Try some peer tutoring—this is where you and a fellow student agree to study together and alternate teaching each other the material. One of you is the instructor, the other the student. Then reverse these roles with each tutoring session.

✓ Work as a team with more organized people. Working around or with

The Healthy Student

Besides contributing to your overall health, the following two suggestions can enhance your academic performance:

1. Watch the caffeine and nicotine use. You're more prone than other students to use these substances and become dependent on them. Adults with ADHD sometimes try to self-medicate their disorder using readily available caffeine-containing beverages or tobacco products. Yes, caffeine and nicotine are stimulants and can help people be more alert. But caffeine, especially, works on the wrong brain neurochemicals for people with ADHD and can, in moderate or high doses, be counterproductive, making you less focused, more jumpy and jittery, more nervous, and more likely to need to urinate frequently. You are better off using a prescription ADHD drug than trying to use caffeine-containing substances or over-the-counter pills that contain this substance. And, while nicotine may benefit your ADHD symptoms to some degree, you're using a highly addictive drug to self-medicate, one that is only going to increase your addiction to this chemical, not to mention increasing your risk for pulmonary and heart disease and cancer. Again, use a prescription ADHD drug instead that does not carry such risks and works just as well or even better.

2. Develop a regular weekly exercise routine (three or more times per week) for increased attention, better health, stress management, and so forth. Regular routine physical exercise done three to four times per week, even for just 20–30 minutes each time, is good for anyone's health. But if you have ADHD, it also seems to be of particular benefit in further controlling your symptoms or compensating for them. So whether it's running, biking, weight training, dance classes, using your favorite gym equipment (such as treadmills, elliptical trainers, stair-climbers), or some mixture of various types of exercise, you, more than most people, need to be doing routine physical exercise.

others who do not have ADHD can keep you better focused on the work and more publicly accountable for doing that work than going solo.

✓ Find a fall-back college classmate who will fill you in if you've forgotten an assignment or other important information. Swap phone numbers and e-mail addresses so that you can get the lost or missing information quickly when you find yourself in a jam.

✓ Attend any after-class help sessions that are offered. Many teachers are willing to set aside extra time to help people who need more instruction. Take teachers up on these offers even if you don't really need the assistance. The extra review will help with your forgetfulness, and it will also show you're motivated, which will make a better impression on your instructors.

✓ Schedule faculty or adviser review meetings often—every 3–6 weeks. Remember that the more often you're held accountable for your work, the better you'll do.

25

Work

"I was so active as a child, my teachers used to tell my mother to 'just keep her busy' because I was always getting into things if I was left alone or without anything to do. I still find it very difficult to stay seated for very long, especially during boring meetings or when I have to do work that doesn't interest me. I just have to be doing something, and if there is anything more interesting or fun to do than the work I've been assigned, I'm likely to get distracted by it and find myself not getting things done on time."

"I have to put in five to ten times more effort at work to do what other people seem to do so easily. By the end of the day at work, I'm exhausted and haven't accomplished half of what other people seem to have done that day. Yet I seem to be more tired than they are. What's with me, anyway?"

"I'm in my mid-30s and have a long-held belief that I may be affected by adult attention deficit disorder of the predominantly inattentive type. I have long suffered a feeling of being different, a feeling that something is not right with me. For a while I thought I may have ADHD, but I'm not fidgety or restless, though I find it very difficult to concentrate and focus on any kind of task assigned to me. While this resulted in much lower grades than I believed I was capable of in school and a feeling that I was 'just not that smart,' it has affected me in a much more serious way during my working life. I am very disorganized and frequently make careless and silly mistakes at work (as I am a mechanical engineer, these can be very costly financially and in regard to my own safety). I struggle to follow instructions, forget where I have put things, and in general have trouble paying attention. These things have led me to feel like a failure at work, and after several attempts to leave my area of work I have embarked on other pursuits that have ended in the same feeling of hopelessness and failure."

Back in the 1990s, research that looked at how ADHD affected teenagers at work concluded that they did pretty much as well as other teenagers. Maybe, it seemed, the symptoms interfered mainly in educational settings and we didn't need to worry so much about jobs.

We now know that's not true. As attested by the last quote above, ADHD can hurt you even *more* at work than it has at school. The problem with those 25-year-old studies is that they failed to take into account the types of jobs adolescents usually hold: unskilled, part-time, and temporary. Working at a local rec center, fast-food joint, or car wash doesn't demand a lot of attention, thought, or persistence. Maybe ADHD really *wouldn't* interfere much in those entry-level occupations.

But when scientists looked at the transition to full-time jobs, a different picture began to emerge. Adults with ADHD were found to change jobs more often and to have more trouble meeting the demands of their jobs, working independently, finishing tasks, and getting along with the boss. They were fired or laid off more often than adults without ADHD.

The adults who had the biggest problems with ADHD in the workplace were those who were hyperactive. Makes sense, doesn't it? Teachers might cut you some slack for being fidgety and restless at school because you're either a growing little kid or a hormone-fired teenager. Once you're in the workplace, those who are paying you to be there expect you to stay at your desk or machinery or other workstation to get your work done. Employees who can't are often labeled slackers and eventually let go.

How much ADHD hinders you at work may depend on the severity of your symptoms, whether they include hyperactivity as just noted, how little emotional control you manifest, and whether you're getting the treatment that the engineer quoted above wasn't. It can also depend on factors like these:

✓ The type of work you do

✓ Whether you're getting any accommodations or supports on the job

✓ How much ADHD prevented you from building the skills and knowledge as a child that we all need in the adult world

Finding the Right Job for You

It's important to have a job where you get as much of what you need to succeed as you possibly can:

✓ Are there jobs you should favor over others because of your symptoms?

✓ Is one type of workplace better for you than others?

✓ Is the work you'll do as important as the environment in which you'll be doing it?

These are questions you should try to answer whether you're just entering the workforce or you already have a job. Naturally there are no easy answers. (Sorry.) But you'll be on the right track if you start by knowing what you're up against and also what you have to offer. If your ADHD includes hyperactivity, a job that requires you to plant yourself in a chair in front of a computer all day is not likely to be ideal. You might toss out any thoughts of becoming an accountant. If your downfall is not being able to finish even short tasks without close supervision, you won't want to become a lone wolf traveling salesperson or a telecommuter working from a home office.

But these are points to consider more than they are firm rules. I know many adults with ADHD who have chosen a job or a field that on the surface doesn't seem ideal for the strengths and weaknesses normally associated with the condition or with their particular version of it. Yet they do as well as most people. How? They get support from a supervisor. They've been given the go-ahead and the resources to adapt the workplace and working procedures to their needs. They demonstrate a commitment to building their skills, using principles like the rules in Step Four and strategies like those you'll find in this chapter. They have a strong inherent love for the type of work they chose to do. They take medication that greatly reduces the impact of their symptoms—particularly critical if hyperactivity or impulsivity is a problem for you.

The engineer whose story you heard at the beginning of this chapter may have chosen what seemed like the best type of work for himself. He may have been attracted to engineering because of a strength in math and graphics—seeing and manipulating objects instead of reading words. Maybe he knew that this is the type of work that absorbs him. If your ADHD sometimes makes it hard for you to wrench yourself away from activities you enjoy, choosing one of those activities for your career is not a bad approach.

Unfortunately, this engineer couldn't succeed. Maybe that was because doing well in a job is never just about the work you do. It also has to do with getting along with your boss and your coworkers. It involves having a physical environment that's conducive to focusing despite the distractibility of ADHD. It depends on your knowing what types of tasks and situations are hardest for you and adapting them so you can deal with them. It may also hinge on whether the work hours overlap with your most alert periods of the day. That may mean finding a sympathetic, supportive organization that will accommodate your needs to some extent. But it most certainly means taking responsibility for using the resources available to you outside of what the company is willing to offer and making a commitment to owning and working with your ADHD.

Our engineer said he couldn't concentrate on conversations and couldn't form lasting, healthy relationships. Undoubtedly that made it hard for him to cultivate cooperation among his coworkers and to enlist the aid of his supervisor in identifying and preventing those "silly mistakes" he was always making. Maybe he also worked in a busy, noisy office that made it hard to focus. Perhaps he didn't have the storage space to organize his materials so he wouldn't forget things.

Because he hasn't been diagnosed with ADHD, this engineer can't officially request accommodations (and isn't receiving the benefit of medication). But he might have found an engineering job at a smaller company or looked for a generally subdued environment. He might have looked for an office designed with private, relatively soundproof workspaces. A company that would pair him up with an assistant or partner who could do the face-to-face contact work for him might have spared him the embarrassment of communication gaffes.

Realistically, we can't all pick and choose among a number of job opportunities, especially if the job market happens to be tight. That's why it's important to map as many different routes to success as you can. Know what type of work might keep you interested and be doable every day. Figure out what type of environment is one in which you're likely to thrive. Know what types of work procedures will keep you on track and which ones will throw you off. Figure out what types of people will inspire, and possibly help, you to succeed. Then do your best to find as many of these favorable elements as you can in any job you consider. For most adults with ADHD, finding the right job will be a matter of identifying the right mix of the work you do (including the procedures) *and* the environment (including the people) you'll be doing it in. Challenges in one can be offset by benefits in the other.

The way many people find such a match is, unfortunately, through trial and error. That process can be painful if it doesn't lead fairly quickly to a good fit. *So another route to consider is to find a professional life coach or vocational counselor who works with people who have ADHD.* This person can at least help you define your needs accurately. A coach can also help you identify lines of work that might be good for you. And a coach can train you in job interviewing—research has shown that adults with ADHD don't interview as well as other adults either.

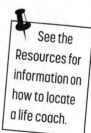

See the Resources for information on how to locate a life coach.

The Type of Work

Some jobs are by nature more ADHD-friendly than others. For instance, these occupations have proven better for some of my adult patients and may be ADHD-friendlier than others:

✓ **The military**—The military ensures greater structure and discipline, more immediate feedback, and greater provision of benefits (like medical care and dental care) than other fields.

✓ **Door-to-door (or B-to-B) sales**—This type of job is often a good fit for adults with ADHD, whether it is door to door, direct to consumer, or business to business. That is because it involves freedom of movement, changes in setting, mobility, a flexible schedule, frequent meetings with new contacts, opportunities for social interaction, and passion for the product, and a value is put on being talkative. Often adults with ADHD need some assistance back at the home office with completing reports and paperwork, but while "in the field" they seem to do well.

✓ **Drug rep**—Individuals with at least a BA degree in biology, nursing, medicine, pharmaceuticals, or a related field may find this calling perfect for all of the same reasons given for door-to-door sales.

✓ **Carpenter, plumber, electrician, landscaper, tile layer, roofer, construction contractor**—These and other trades may be more ADHD-friendly because the individual is doing more manual than mental work, is outdoors more often, has frequent changes in job sites, gets to deal with a lot of different people, and is paid an hourly wage, which provides for more immediate consequences than a salaried position with its less frequent paycheck.

✓ **Emergency medical technician, emergency room physician, police officer, firefighter**—Like the jobs above, these occupations do not keep people confined to offices or require hours of sustained mental effort or concentration. They also provide some excitement and thrills, and even life-threatening situations that can provide the burst of adrenaline some adults with ADHD claim helps them focus their mind in a crisis. Again, greater freedom of movement, changes in work settings, and greater interaction with others may combine with the sensation-producing nature of these jobs to make them more friendly to those with ADHD. It is not that people with ADHD are better than others at handling crises, but that in a crisis the person with ADHD is at no disadvantage because there is little or no preparation needed to deal with the situation—after all, that is the definition of a crisis (an unexpected yet serious event).

✓ **Sports**—Some talented athletes have found that ADHD does not exact a big price for success. Think about Olympic swimmer Michael Phelps, late pro golfer Payne Stewart, and Olympic gymnast Simone Biles. Becoming a professional athlete is not in the cards for most of us, but there are many other sports-related occupations, from phys ed teacher and school sports coach to jobs at outdoor sports parks and health clubs, personal trainer jobs and jobs teaching others your sport, and even ranger jobs at national and state parks.

✓ **Computer technician/consultant**—Here your computer knowledge and skills can coexist with your ADHD traits with less impairment than in other fields. Those working on the IT "help desk" rove throughout a business, resolving computer issues for other employees.

✓ **Food service industry**—I know many adults with ADHD who have gone into culinary arts and become chefs at restaurants, resorts, cafeterias, and other places of employment and found the work to be creative and relatively unaffected by their ADHD-related deficits. Cooking requires a focus on the moment, the immediate steps to create the finished product, and a flair for creativity with ingredients while not demanding long-range planning, lots of working memory, or persistence at unrewarding activities for long periods of time. Unusual or flexible hours, with the sporadic ebb-and-flow pacing of the work from slow to peak meal-prep hours and then slow again, can add just the right touch of crisis and excitement during the peak meal hours to keep you alert and focused on the work at hand.

✓ **Self-employment/entrepreneurship**—Starting a small business or just being a sole proprietor can prove ADHD-friendly, whether you open your own bakery, run a landscaping, computer consulting, or personal fitness coaching business, or work in one of the trades listed above. The hours can be more flexible than when you work with others, you are your own boss, the consequences for working (or not working) are immediate (no work, no food or rent money), and the work settings can vary considerably from day to day, accommodating the restlessness that many adults with ADHD experience. One notch up from being self-employed in an established field, such as landscaping, home building, housecleaning, or running a restaurant or car wash, is being an entrepreneur. The term usually refers to people who create new products, services, or even entire industries in innovative ways that carry a greater financial risk but also a greater payoff than most other self-employment. Johan Wiklund, an endowed chair in the entrepreneurial studies division of the School of Business at Syracuse University, believes that entrepreneurs are more likely to have ADHD and are more likely to succeed because of it, particularly if they are highly intelligent and have little or no comorbid (additional) psychiatric disorders. Their disinhibited and hence more creative thought process, willingness to take risks, hyperfocusing on work they love, and engaging social styles may all combine to make for entrepreneurial success.

✓ **Photographer/videographer**—Many of the adults who assisted me in creating my various DVDs on ADHD or with whom I have worked on various media projects were themselves adults with the disorder. They were able to deal quite well with the day-to-day changes in settings where they would be filming, the diversity of stories or topics they were asked to cover, the short bursts of work interspersed with breaks, and, of course, the frequent opportunities to interact with a variety of people, all of which were a good fit for their short attention span, propensity for boredom in tedious environments, and difficulties with sustained effort across hours or days and projects or tasks.

✓ **Performing arts**—Actors, comedians, musicians, and others in the performing arts often rely on emotional expression and can take advantage of frequent changes in the setting and nature of the work, freedom of movement, limited need for long-range planning and organization, and low requirement for self-motivation given the immediate and intrinsic pleasure people may get from engaging in these professions. Howie Mandel (*America's Got Talent*) has ADHD yet has been quite successful in comedy and show business; Ty Pennington (*Extreme Makeover: Home Edition*) likewise has adult ADHD yet has served as the central character in a show that has done much good for needy families. And so does Glenn Beck, former Fox News commentator and now independent radio show host. Also consider musician Adam Levine, lead singer/songwriter of Maroon 5 and former judge on TV's *The Voice*.

These are just some examples of occupations that may prove to be especially friendly to those having ADHD. If you use the descriptions as a springboard for your imagination, you can undoubtedly come up with other career paths that would be suitable for you given your own set of unique aptitudes and flair for the nontraditional avenues of work. But you also need to consider the working environment.

The Working Environment

✓ Do noise and other distractions keep you from focusing no matter what the work is? If so, an open room full of desks could be a disaster for you. Even bays that have clusters with a smaller number of desks might be a problem because it will be tough to block out your coworkers. Cubicles with opaque walls that keep you from noticing the movement of passersby are better. A private office might be best of all if you can get it. The ideal would be a workspace away from the main traffic pattern but close to your supervisor or other person to whom you'll be accountable. If you have an office, keep the door closed. If necessary because of office noise, use Bluetooth noise-canceling headphones and listen to your favorite instrumental music while working. If someone happens by, meet the person at the door and lean against the jamb so he or she doesn't waltz in and take a seat just to visit. Don't offer coffee or food, but be gracious and ask immediately how you can help the person. Coworkers can be huge sources of distraction or "off-task" activities, so limit such interference when you can.

✓ Will you be working at a computer with e-mail? If so, and your job doesn't depend on rapid response to e-mails, resolve to check it briefly at the beginning of the day for urgent messages from supervisors or coworkers, then shut off the e-mail program and don't check it again until lunch and then again at the end of the day. This gives you more time in the middle of the morning and afternoon to focus on the projects you need to tackle and eliminates one of the greatest sources of distraction and low productivity in the workplace.

✓ Is the Internet available? Keep your Internet browser closed as well so that pop-up ads, chimes, or other attention-getting stimuli cannot disrupt your concentration on the projects that need your attention. And definitely avoid text messaging or tweeting friends or others during the workday by shutting down your cell phone for periods when your concentration on tasks or projects is important. As with e-mail, you can check your phone messages two to three times per day (beginning, middle, end) and keep up with anything that may be urgent and important. But most e-mails and, especially, text messages are not relevant to your immediate work and often are just attempts to socialize by others who cannot focus on their work either.

✓ Will your assigned space help you get organized? If there's no room for you to put your files and other materials, you could spend the majority of your workday looking for what you need.

✓ Will you be able to keep track of the passing hours? If you have no windows, no wall clocks, and no other way to tell what time it is, you'll have to rely solely on your own tools to keep track of the time and stay on schedule. That can be hard for adults with ADHD, who cannot seem to harness their internal clocks to keep them functioning in a timely manner. If you are on a computer, most have clock apps that you can open and show the passage of time to help you with this. E-mail services and calendar or other organizing apps can help you with alerts that you program into them when you initially set up certain goals, meetings, trips, or other projects in them. The alarm function in your smartphone can achieve the same result by pinging you every so often as a reminder to stay focused on the task at hand.

Work Procedures

✓ How much flexibility is there? Sometimes a job interview instantly reveals that the company expects the job to be done in a very specific way and has no resources available for bending the way things have been done in the past. Always ask questions about how the hirer will expect the goals to be met:

- "How long would you expect X to take to get done?"

- "How much advance notice will I have of an upcoming project?"

- "How often would I check in with you on my progress?"

- "In what form would you expect to receive reports?"

- "Will I be working on my own or with a team?"

Beware the interviewer who says it's a "very loose" kind of operation and that everyone can get the job done in the best way for the employee with little or no supervision. Ask questions like the preceding and you may quickly find out that there are actually much stricter requirements than the person has let on. Or, if you don't ask for specifics, you might find out on the job that "loose" is an understatement and that you're expected to be completely self-sufficient. This may make it tough to introduce the idea of making yourself accountable to someone for step-by-step progress on tasks.

✓ Are there established "rules" or guidelines for certain procedures? Most adults with ADHD benefit from having a set of rules to follow so that they don't have to try to figure out what's acceptable and what's not. If this firm hasn't established such rules, will a supervisor or mentor be available to clarify priorities when you're new at the job?

✓ Will you be expected to be a self-starter? You might find that overwhelming and would want to steer clear of jobs like this. Or you might find it's easy to be a self-starter but harder to be a self-motivator once a task is under way. Which leads to the next question:

✓ Does the job offer built-in frequent incentives and rewards? The more, the better. Virtue may be its own reward for other people, but ADHD says, "Show me the money" . . . and on a regular basis. If there are no opportunities for motivating you other than those you provide yourself, find another job—or resolve to collect every type of external cue and reward at your disposal.

✓ Do you have to punch a time clock, literally or figuratively? My research has shown that adults with ADHD tend to be less punctual for work and appear to manage their time less efficiently. If strict work hours and punctuality are essential or time is of the essence in this business, it may prove to be your doom. Or, all else being favorable, you could choose to turn this to your advantage and make it all part of your commitment to keeping track of time.

The People

✓ Who will be your supervisor?

- Someone you'll work with every day, face-to-face?

- Someone you'll be expected to report to throughout the day remotely (by e-mail or phone)?

- Someone you'll rarely see at all who will occasionally just send you a list of objectives?

You're likely to need a fair amount of hands-on oversight and interaction. If your supervisor won't be able to give you much guidance or keep you accountable, is someone else available to do that and serve as a mentor?

✓ Will your supervisor be supportive of what you need to get the job done? Whether the job can be adapted to suit your needs often depends largely on your supervisor. If your boss takes a sink-or-swim attitude with employees and doesn't give a hoot about individual needs, you should probably find another job.

✓ Will your coworkers be supportive too? Or will you be swimming with sharks? If this business's approach to reaching goals or achieving excellence is to pit employees against each other in cutthroat competition, can you handle it? Some adults with ADHD have developed a heightened sensitivity to the responses they get from others. Given good reason to believe your coworkers are out to get you, will you be inspired to beat them, or will you find it impossible to get your work done?

 Should I reveal that I have ADHD when I'm interviewing for a job?

If you're going to assert your right to receive workplace accommodations under the Americans with Disabilities Act, yes. You may have to invoke that law to get what you need. If you are going to work in a field that requires periodic training, testing, or certification, you may need special accommodations for test taking, available through the act. In that case you'll have to provide paperwork to document your diagnosis. But you may be able to get what you need just by finding the right type of workplace. This is why it's so important to ask the questions listed above. If you can tell that the company and your supervisor will be flexible and supportive without your having to name your disorder, you may be able to keep that information private. Many adults prefer not to disclose their ADHD. And you might not have to if you do everything in your power to minimize your symptoms. This is another reason to avail yourself of medication. If it normalizes or greatly reduces your symptoms, ADHD won't need to come up at all.

Laying the Groundwork for Success on the Job

If you haven't read Chapter 24, you might want to skim it even if you're not in school for full details about some of the tools and tips listed there.

Many of the tools and preparation steps for doing well at work parallel those for doing well at school. Here's a quick rundown of what you can do to give yourself the best possible foundation for occupational achievement:

✔ Consult one of the books listed in the Resources at the back of this book to familiarize yourself with the provisions of the Americans with Disabilities Act and the accommodations typically available in the workplace. You may want to avail yourself of these accommodations at some point even if not right now.

✔ Practice, practice, practice the strategies under the eight everyday rules for success given in Step Four. When you're considering taking a particular job, think about how these rules might benefit you in that workplace. As recommended there, make a list and post these in your office or near your computer screen so you can refer to them frequently throughout the day.

✔ Consider medication if you aren't already taking it. This may be especially helpful if you're making the transition from the less demanding jobs of adolescence to the adult jobs that require a lot more time, effort, achievement, responsibility, and skills. As with school, the long-acting forms (sometimes with a single dose of the immediate-release medicine added later in the day) will keep you going through most of the workday.

✔ Find a coach or mentor at work. This can be a coworker, friend, or supportive supervisor—anyone you can make yourself accountable to every day for the work that you believe needs to get done. As with school, it helps to meet twice a day for 5 minutes at a time—which is why it's useful to have your supervisor or

Recruiting a coach/mentor is critical and can benefit you far beyond the accountability it will provide. If you gain this person's respect, others will hear about it, and you may find yourself with allies you didn't actively cultivate. So make it a priority to do what you've agreed to do with your coach or mentor. Show your appreciation through small tokens of thanks. Resist any urge to seek this person's advice or help with personal problems; stick to company business. (You can always see a life coach if you need help with personal issues.)

other coach in close proximity. Set goals during your first meeting and then review what you've accomplished during the second meeting.

✓ Identify the disability specialist in the human resources department at your company. This is the person you will provide with documentation of your ADHD and the person who will explain the available workplace accommodations. This person may also work with your supervisor to make sure you get the accommodations you choose. If you need therapy or medication, the disability specialist will be able to refer you to psychologists, counselors, and physicians (usually psychiatrists) who have contracts with the employer for providing employee mental health services.

✓ Gather whatever tools will help you keep track of tasks, goals, deadlines, promises, appointments, and any other time-related information you need to remember:

- Day planners

- Smartphones

- Your journal

- The calendar in your e-mail system

- A tactile cueing device such as the MotivAider (see *amazon.com*), or the timers on your smartphone, which can be set to vibrate at certain intervals or at random to remind you to stay on task

> See Chapter 19 for more on using a journal. I can't stress enough how critical your journal is to success in all domains of your life.

✓ Get a recorder such as the Smartpen digital recorder (see *livescribe.com*) to record important meetings (with the permission of your supervisor).

Reclaiming the Edge That ADHD Tries to Take Away

There's no denying that it's a competitive world. If you don't do well at your job, you won't get a raise or promotion. You might not even get to keep the job. And there's always someone waiting in line to claim it. It's also human nature to want to achieve and excel and be respected by our peers. So, do everything you can to be at the top of your game at work despite ADHD.

✓ Find out if there is a library or information center that contains resources for further learning on the job. If so, you'll want to make a habit of using it to give yourself the informational edge that ADHD dulls. Also attend any extra information sessions offered after hours. And if a seminar or workshop is offered on a volunteer basis, volunteer to go. It may sound boring, but a change of scene may be even more beneficial to you than to most adults.

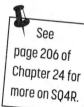

See pages 205–206 of Chapter 24 for tips on staying on your game by being fit.

✓ Take notes throughout meetings that threaten to bore you to tears. Note taking may remind you of some of your least favorite moments in school, but laptops and tablets make it easy to record what's going on, especially if they have a handwriting recognition tablet or screen, and the sheer physical motion of taking notes will keep you focused—to say nothing of providing a great resource that you can refer to later if you're having trouble re-creating what everyone said.

✓ Use the SQ4R method when you have lots of reading to do before a meeting or other event.

✓ Walk around the block or the halls or come up with an excuse to go down to the convenience store or coffee bar in the lobby or around the corner before a long meeting or other quiet period where you'll have to stay seated and be attentive. A brisk walk of just a few minutes will improve your concentration for about an hour afterward.

See page 206 of Chapter 24 for more on SQ4R.

Cultivating Allies at Work

Step Two explained why good relationships with others often elude adults with ADHD. Limited self-regulation can make social interactions challenging. The mere fact that you've been exposed to a lot of criticism, possibly for most of your life, can make you touchy and overcautious in approaching people for help or friendship. For this reason you might not be facile at recruiting allies and friendly colleagues. You might butt heads with your boss. Yet it's widely known today that success at work (and everywhere else) can be as much a function of social skills and savoir faire as it is of practical skills, knowledge, intelligence, and drive. Here are some specific ideas for cultivating the cooperation, compassion, and goodwill of your coworkers. These ideas will not only make your workday more pleasant but will get you an edge in meeting the demands of your job.

- Try some cooperative coworker tutoring when you need to learn something substantial on the job: new software, new regulatory codes, new legislation, new technology—whatever you need to master to keep performing well in the job. Maybe each of you reads a chapter of a new manual and then explains it to the other.

- If your department doesn't already operate using teams, set one up on your own. Be on the lookout for the coworkers who have the skills and interests you lack. Figure out what you can offer that is not a strength of theirs. Identify a departmental goal that you can achieve faster and better working together than you could singly.

- Find a coworker who will have your back—and do the same for that person. If either of you forgets materials, information, or anything else you need while away from the office, the other will be there to supply it. This can be a boon if you don't have secretaries or assistants and you need information not available via computer when you're traveling for business.

- Be fair and reasonable when you request support and accommodations from your supervisor, the disability specialist, and even coworkers who have shown a willingness to help you out. One person I know said she found it just as helpful that her human resources contact would tell her straight out what the company could *not* do to accommodate her needs as what it *could* do. The parameters had been drawn clearly, and the employee kept these limitations in mind whenever she felt tempted to ask for more help than she was getting. Mutual respect resulted.

- Schedule supervisor review meetings more often than at annual or semiannual performance/salary review meetings. Every 3 to 6 weeks is a good interval to aim for. The person you meet with may not be your direct supervisor but someone further up the ladder who can give you another perspective on how you're doing. Who this person would be depends on the structure of your company. Requests you make for this feedback may not be met by the person you ask first, but any higher-up will respect your desire to monitor and better your performance.

26

Money

"Things like balancing my checkbook, paying traffic tickets, getting regular dental checkups, and other routine things seem to elude me. But, hey, I finally pay the rent and utility bills on time, so that's a victory. I haven't had my utilities shut down for nonpayment for quite a while."

When you have ADHD, there's a money pit everywhere you turn. Any opportunity to spend can turn into an impulse purchase. Money problems among adults with ADHD run the gamut from overspending to nonpayment of bills to failure to plan for retirement.

Our research has found that adults with ADHD:

- Made a lot of impulse purchases
- Had high credit card balances
- Exceeded their credit limits more than others
- Made bill, loan, and rent payments late or not at all
- Had their cars repossessed more often than others
- Had lower credit ratings
- Were more likely to have no savings
- Were less likely to save for retirement
- Bounced checks more often than others
- Often failed to save receipts that could document money-saving tax deductions and other documents for their income tax returns
- Lost friends after borrowing money and not repaying it

If you are like most adults with ADHD, you've experienced a lot of these problems. You probably understand why the woman quoted above thought not having her utilities turned off was a major achievement. Money trouble can permeate—even rule—your life, and it's a lot harder to get out of than it is to get into. And there are so many different ways money can be a trap for you—any one financial problem has a way of spawning a number of others. Exceed your credit limit or pile up too much student debt and pay your bills late often enough and your credit rating plummets. You could easily be denied a mortgage or a car loan when you need one. Continuing to pay rent or having to live with a clunker that needs constant costly repairs can absorb your paycheck, leaving you nothing to save. Then what do you do when you suddenly have a car accident and need to pay the deductibles on both your health insurance and car insurance and have no cash?

Money problems are also notorious for causing relationship conflict. Trying to extricate yourself from debt may lead to borrowing money and alienating those who now feel the burden of your financial trouble. Disputes with intimate partners often center on money matters, and they may get even more heated when one person has trouble managing money due to ADHD.

Why Money Matters Are So Challenging for You . . . and What You Can Do about It

If, like many adults with ADHD, you've ended up in financial trouble, it's not necessarily that you don't wish to be solvent or that you don't understand how to get there. But ADHD has a way of letting your best intentions and your knowledge fall by the wayside. Fortunately, you can take charge of your ADHD *and* your finances. The deficits caused by ADHD can steer you wrong, but you can steer yourself back in the right direction:

Money and the Mind's Eye

Impulsive shopping can become compulsive shopping when your nonverbal working memory is weak. You can't picture what happened last time you bought an expensive item you didn't need. You can't bring the future into sharp enough relief to put off the purchase till you've saved the cash. You haven't developed the self-awareness to realize that for you walking into an antique store is like opening the gates of hell. The mind's eye is particularly important in controlling the impulse to buy things you don't need or can't afford.

See more on how the mind's eye works in Chapter 9 and how to make the most of it in Chapter 17.

Using strategies from Step Four, you could externalize the desire to resist spending money by keeping a photo of a long-term goal (a vacation spot, a home, a bike for one of your kids, and so forth) in your pocket to pull out whenever you feel the urge to buy. You might train yourself to say out loud before you pull out your wallet, "Hmmmm, do I really need this?" Or put a sticky note on your credit card that simply says, "NO!" Then you could turn on your imaginary wide-screen TV and watch a film of yourself opening your credit card bill the last time you overspent.

Your Finances and the Mind's Voice

Remember, the mind's voice is your backup when the mind's eye is myopic. If you find yourself feeling the urge to pull out your credit card and you really can't call up a visual picture of what happened the last time you overspent, interview yourself. If you're in a store, leave and do this on the sidewalk. As I mentioned in Step Four, you won't get hauled away for being delusional; people will just think you're on your cell phone when you talk to yourself about whether this purchase or withdrawal is wise. Consider asking a friend to serve as a gatekeeper for your purchases—someone you will text or call before making any purchase so that he or she can ask whether you really need this item and hold you accountable for your spending. Offer to reciprocate.

If you tend to put off bill paying even when you've set an alarm to remind you to do it, this is another time you can talk to yourself about why you need to do it right now. The mind's voice is also the faculty that allows you to formulate and use rules. Set certain rules about spending and saving and then repeat those rules to yourself quietly when under pressure from your ADHD to break them. Or write them down on a card you keep banded together with your credit card so you can't access the credit card without the rules card.

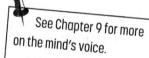

See Chapter 9 for more on the mind's voice.

See Chapter 18 for more on training the mind's voice.

See Chapter 19 for tools you can use to remind yourself to save and not spend.

If forgetting is the main reason you don't pay bills on time, all of the reminder devices discussed in Step Four, plus your journal, can provide you with the necessary cues.

The Mind's Heart in the World of Money

Are you an emotional spender? Are you the person who always buys a round of drinks at the pub when you're feeling great? The one who "needs" a new outfit when you feel down? If you're mad at your landlord, do you "show him" by "forgetting" to pay the rent? Does not having the cash to go out with friends make you feel so bad that you decide to put the charges on your credit card? You're going to have to pull out your whole bag of mental imagery and self-talk tricks to recognize when your emotions are carrying you away and how to get control. Also try to stick to a healthy lifestyle. Sleep deprivation, overconsumption of caffeine or alcohol, drug use, lack of exercise, and poor diet can all make you more vulnerable to daily stress and make it harder to control your emotions.

See Chapter 9 for more on the mind's heart and Chapter 20 for ways to use your emotions to motivate you to handle your finances the way you want to.

Don't forget that you can use your emotions for good too. Hate bill paying? Feel the future: Do everything you can to feel the relief of getting it done. Can't motivate yourself to put money in savings when your paycheck is burning a hole in your pocket? Set up automatic deposits through work so you don't see the money at all. Feel how great it will be to take it out when you pay for your Caribbean vacation.

Financial Planning and Problem Solving in the Mind's Playground

Many adults, ADHD or no ADHD, just don't know how to do financial planning, budget, oversee their investments, or keep track of income and expenditures. If this is true for you, try making money matters physical, as emphasized in Step Four.

See Chapter 9 for more on the mind's playground and Chapter 22 to get ideas for making money management tangible.

Use tangible objects and graphic tools to manipulate the numbers whenever possible. The following pages will give you some ideas. But remember the basics too: Make lists of steps to complete financial tasks you find daunting. Record your spending habits in your journal so you can take a look back at the patterns that are hurting you and any that are serving you well.

Getting Control of Your Money

Fortunately, you've got a lot of resources at your fingertips for taking back control of your financial present and future. There are many strategies for discouraging spending. Tools and cues can help you meet your financial obligations on time. You can set up systems that enforce saving so you don't have to fight the urge to spend everything you earn over and over. You can even access free credit counseling through certain banks or government programs in some regions.

A New Approach to Money Management

Here are a few ideas for getting started on a better path:

✔ *Take advantage of community resources if you're in trouble.* It's paramount that you become more aware of community resources, such as assistance from banks, credit unions, and others who may be able to help you address these money management problems. Debt reorganization, credit counseling, budgeting advice, and bankruptcy assistance are all available. If you are massively in debt and it seems hopeless or you're thinking of declaring bankruptcy, get free credit counseling first from a bank or credit union. They can often help you reorganize your finances, consolidate debt, and renegotiate unusually high interest rates and meet with you monthly to keep you and your budget on track and keep you accountable to someone besides yourself.

✔ *Let your spouse, partner, or even parent manage your money.* Doing this presumes this person does not also have ADHD and can be trusted to manage your finances with your best interests in mind. It might be something to consider if you feel overwhelmed by the problems you're having and find it impossible to control your spending or other financial habits. You can always agree to do this for a preset temporary time period or until a certain goal—such as paying off a debt or accumulating a certain amount of savings—is reached. Turn over your paycheck to this person, let the person allocate sufficient cash to you to meet daily expenses, then work together to see that monthly bills, loans, and credit cards are paid regularly. If appropriate, have your manager set up an automatic bill-paying system with your bank so that some important bills like rent, mortgage, and car loan payments are automatically deducted from your checking account each month. And don't forget to reward your helper periodically, such as with lunch out, a takeout meal, or an Internet coffee shop or restaurant gift card, or just bake some cookies or brownies occasionally.

✔ *Budget!* Make a monthly budget sheet that shows *all* your monthly expenses, including one-twelfth of your annual expenses (those that you may pay just once per year, such as taxes, car insurance, and homeowner's insurance). You need to have a monthly financial plan with all your bills listed in front of you so you can see what you owe. This budget needs to be less than what you make per month. Keep

> You can get software programs to help with setting up a budget, but I favor good old-fashioned pencil and paper—just as easy and cheaper.

it out on your desk at home where you do paperwork or on your dresser so you can refer to it often. Spending as you go each month is a recipe for disaster, not to mention having your utilities turned off and your car repossessed.

> **Unexpected medical costs are one of the biggest sources of unanticipated expenses, large debts, and even bankruptcy.**

✓ *Start living within your means* **today.** Do not spend more each month than you earn and then try to use credit cards, loans, or other means of borrowing to see you through the month. You need to get your living expenses below 90% of your monthly earnings while saving that remaining 10%. Enlist the help of a competent, trusted relative, an accountant, or a bank employee in figuring out your expenses and what method is best for saving.

✓ *Set up a system of accounts and deposits for enforced savings.* Have your employer put 10% of your pretax earnings into a retirement plan (tax deferred) such as a 401(k), 403(b), Keogh, or IRA. Often they will match your contribution up to a certain amount. That is free money you are leaving on the table if you don't take advantage of these plans at work when they are available. Then have your after-tax paycheck direct deposited into your checking account. Once it is there, have your bank move 10% of it into a savings account automatically each month. The less you see of your cash, the less you can spend it impulsively. You also need an emergency savings account to cover unexpected expenses such as car repairs and medical expenses not covered by insurance. If that does not leave you enough

> **If you don't save at least 10% of your income, you are having your vacation/retirement *now* and will be working the rest of your life to pay for it!**

for your usual monthly expenses, cut down on those expenses instead. You can find enough fat in your budget to cut your expenses by 10% so you can start saving. Many people find, for example, that brewing their own coffee and taking homemade lunches to work instead of patronizing coffee shops and restaurants builds daily savings that really add up.

✓ *Try to get health and disability insurance through your employer.* Always assess such benefits when looking for a job, and keep in mind that government employers at all levels nearly always provide these benefits.

✓ *Balance your bank statement monthly without fail.* Don't just wing it or guess. Having little idea of how much money you have in your account(s) at any one time is one of the biggest causes of credit card overuse, overdrafts, and debt accumulation. Keep in mind that many of the new online banks offer no-fee accounts in response to widespread objections to high overdraft and other banking fees, and these banks may offer mobile apps that help you stay on top of your bank balances to the minute.

✔ *Keep all receipts as you get them.* Put them in your wallet. Make a nightly habit of taking out your wallet and going through it to remove all receipts and put them in a file. You can use this file to help keep track of what you are spending and to store the receipts, which will be very useful for preparing your taxes and getting the most out of your available deductions.

Curbing Your Spending

Besides the ideas for controlling impulse buying described earlier, try these:

✔ *Operate on a cash basis.* Withdraw cash from your checking account only when you absolutely need it. Carry as little with you as possible so you're not tempted to spend it impulsively on stuff you don't need.

✔ *Do NOT carry a credit or ATM card if at all possible.* Get rid of all store credit cards, keep one general card like MasterCard or Visa, and put a sticker on it that reads "For Emergency Use Only." Transfer all unpaid balances on store cards to this single card and work to pay off the balance as soon as you possibly can.

> **The minimum credit card payment is based on a 10-year payoff plan, assuming no extra debt is added to the card—*10 years!***

✔ *Do NOT go to a shopping area if there is nothing you need to buy.* And I mean NEED, not want, to buy. And never meet friends to socialize while browsing. The temptation to buy stuff while wandering through stores can be too great when impulse control is limited by ADHD.

✔ *Don't lend anyone other than your children any money.* Period. And even your children are not a good bet to repay you, so keep those loans limited to educational expenses or necessities, not things like clothing or entertainment. Odds are you will not see that money again. If you give money to someone else, you'd better view it as the gift it most likely will be, not as a loan.

✔ *Stay away from casinos.* They always win. Don't play cards for money, and certainly not more than pennies a hand. Avoid places where impulsive gambling can get the best of you, including Internet gaming websites.

✔ *Take advantage of cognitive-behavioral treatments for impulse buying if no other measures help.* If you find it hard to stop shopping and spending on things you don't need, get professional help from a psychologist or financial counselor.

Getting Control of Credit

Besides paying off credit cards and not carrying them, try these ideas:

✓ *Never borrow money for something you consume, wear,
or use for entertainment* (like flat-screen TVs, iPhones). Borrow just for buying a home, getting a car (maybe), or some other reasonable *investment*.

✓ *Do NOT sign any contracts for credit, loans, or similar commitments without having a money manager—your relative or a professional—review it first* to see if you really need to be doing this.

✓ *Never, ever, ever take out a "payday loan."* The storefront businesses that offer these loans charge interest rates that are so high you will never be able to get out of debt. This is legalized loan sharking. Stay away from it. Period.

27

Relationships

"So my wife tells this psychologist we went to see for marital problems that being married to me is like having another child around the house and she already has three of them and doesn't need a fourth, so that if he cannot help us with our marriage and straighten me out she is gonna leave me! She tells him I can't seem to follow through on anything, that I have projects half finished lying around all over the house, and that I cannot have anything ready when it's supposed to be done. She has taken over the paying of all the bills 'cause when I had that job, we had our phone and electric service shut down twice because I forgot to pay the monthly bills or didn't pay them on time."

"I seem to burn through relationships with others a lot faster than the other women I know. My boyfriends sometimes called me a 'space cadet' because when they were talking to me about things, especially things that meant a lot to them, I was just staring at them, or daydreaming and clearly not listening, or I would just interrupt them to talk about something that just came into my mind. Once I was dating this really nice guy and we were getting really serious about each other and then, on a whim, I met this guy in a bar one night when my girlfriends and I were out partying and I just went back to his apartment and slept with him on an impulse. And my boyfriend heard about it from one of the girls with me that night and that was the end of that relationship. I don't know why I do things like that on an impulse. And I can't seem to concentrate on what others are saying to me for very long or stay committed to a good relationship. I mean, I can be my own worst enemy in my life."

You probably don't need a psychologist to tell you how ADHD and its underlying problem with self-control create social difficulties. The way ADHD stacks the deck against you can hurt more in your personal, social life than anywhere else. If you had the condition as a child, you may still carry the scars of being treated as different or undesirable to be around. Today, you might look enviously at others who seem to make friends without trying . . . who have longtime spouses or partners . . . who can call on parents and siblings and colleagues for company and comfort.

You might be highly aware of the ways ADHD is harming your relationships, but you might not know how. There are three aspects of self-control that can have huge effects on your relationships:

When Emotions Take Control Away from You

The executive function called *emotion regulation* causes lots of trouble for adults with ADHD. Unfortunately, because it doesn't seem connected to more widely known symptoms like inattention and hyperactivity, you might not automatically associate emotional upheaval with the disorder. But adults with ADHD report that problems with managing anger, frustration, and hostility when provoked are just as common as their other symptoms and lead to lots of social conflict.

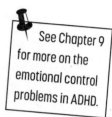
See Chapter 9 for more on the emotional control problems in ADHD.

• • • • • • • • • • • • • • • •
Emotional control problems may make you act boisterous, silly, or melodramatic, but it's uncontrolled anger that threatens your relationships most.
• • • • • • • • • • • • • • • •

Part of what society considers "adult" consists of controlling your temper, dealing quietly with frustration, shrugging off minor slights, managing your impatience while waiting, and shielding others from your moods. So it's hardly surprising that many people will not tolerate emotional outbursts and will often end relationships because of them.

When ADHD Robs You of Self-Awareness

See Rule 2 (Chapter 17) for a couple of strategies you can practice to sharpen your mind's eye so you become more self-aware in the moment.
See *Taking Charge of Anger* (2nd ed.) by W. Robert Nay (Guilford Press, 2012) and *Is It You, Me, or Adult A.D.D.?* by Gina Pera (1201 Alarm Press, 2008) for other methods of anger management.

ADHD diminishes your ability to monitor your ongoing behavior. With hindsight—especially if you've been practicing using your mind's eye—you might be able to see that your emotions can be overwhelming or at least uncomfortable for those in the firing line. You might recognize, ruefully, that some people have opted out of your life because they couldn't stand the heat. *But those revelations don't automatically translate into different behavior at the moment when you're provoked.* Sharpening your hindsight helps, but because emotions are so powerful, awareness might

Our adult patients have often told us that they simply did not realize just how poorly they were coming across to others during social encounters. At least not until it was too late. Some of the social violations they reported committing:

- Dominating conversations with endless monologues or storytelling that went nowhere

- Failing to listen closely for any length of time

- Having trouble reciprocating or taking turns during conversations or social encounters

- Making tactless comments

- Failing to honor social etiquette appropriate to the situation

not be enough to stop the onslaught. Other methods for calming the arousal system in the body can help too.

When ADHD Blurs Life's Scripts

Social encounters with others require more than just the normal give-and-take of conversations or other social actions. Adults have to do a higher level of self-monitoring to know when to start, shift, end, or keep an interaction going. Continuously playing the role of spectator over our own behavior as it plays out with others requires us to perform these steps in every encounter:

Reading entrance and exit cues is just as important as what you do onstage.

1. Read bodily and facial cues

2. Perceive the emotional nuances in tone of voice

3. Adjust our own behavior accordingly

You already know that deficits in executive functions make these steps particularly challenging for you. The ramifications? Every encounter with another person is filled with traps. These traps can exacerbate the problems you already face at work and school with coworkers, classmates, and other casual acquaintances.

They become huge pitfalls in the relationships you want to last, including friendships and particularly closer relationships like intimate partnerships. Let's look at different types of relationships more closely.

Intimate Relationships: Spouses and Partners

The two individuals quoted at the beginning of this chapter poignantly related how ADHD can affect an adult's closest relationships. When one member of a couple has ADHD, the balance of work in the household can end up askew, hurt feelings can result from apparent insensitivity or lack of interest in the other person, and intimacy can be threatened by poorly regulated emotion.

Interestingly, we don't have any evidence that those who grow up with ADHD marry, separate, or divorce more or less often than other adults. That could be, however, because our follow-up studies have gone only as far as ages 20–30—ages at which 55–67% of all adults are still single.

Our research and other studies have shown that adults with ADHD are more likely to have:

- Fair to poor dating relationships (four to five times more likely!).

- Lower-quality marital relationships (our studies found more than a two-fold difference).

- Extramarital affairs.

Keeping ADHD from Ruining Your Closest Relationship

Unfortunately, to date there have been no studies on any particular approach to addressing the problems ADHD can impose on dating and marriage. So I can't offer scientifically based advice. But here are some commonsense ideas flowing from what research we do have:

✓ Get a diagnosis so you can get treatment if you haven't done so already. In working directly with adults, my colleagues and I have seen that medication, by improving symptoms, also improves the relationships between intimate partners.

✓ Read Gina Pera's book *Is It You, Me, or Adult A.D.D.?* (1201 Alarm Press,

2008). This is the best book available right now for partners in relationships where one has adult ADHD. Although the book's advice is largely untested in research studies, it seems sound given what science has revealed about ADHD in adults. The Resources section of this book also includes two volumes on this topic by Melissa Orlov and a book by Ari Tuckman on sex and adult ADHD.

✓ Consider enrolling in a mindfulness meditation class, not so much for any religious training in Buddhism, but for the more secularized mindfulness practices of Jon Kabat-Zinn and others. Multiple recent studies have shown that mindfulness practices can help you cope with the symptoms and executive deficits of adult ADHD, especially those involving emotional control. (For more information see *The Mindfulness Prescription for Adult ADHD* by Lidia Zylowska, described in the Resources.) Mindfulness shows great promise as a supplemental approach to targeting the deficits of adult ADHD alongside medication treatment and cognitive-behavioral therapy, such as that outlined by Mary Solanto in *Cognitive-Behavioral Therapy for Adult ADHD,* listed in the Resources.

✓ Apply the strategies you read about in Step Four. Many couples feel they can be themselves with the person they love. That may be true. But that should mean being your *best* self, someone who tries hard to:

- Think before acting or speaking

- Keep track of what has been hurtful or helpful to the other person in the past

- Remember significant dates like birthdays and anniversaries, using the same kinds of external cues you use to remind yourself of doctors' appointments, work deadlines, and other obligations

- *Listen*

- Exercise tact, kindness, and courtesy

- Do a fair share of household chores

- Be a good parent if you have kids, which leads us to . . .

• • • • • • • • • •
Adults with ADHD report much higher parental stress than other parents.
• • • • • • • • • •

Parenting

Parenting is the most stressful role that many of us play in life. ADHD ups the ante in these ways, among others:

✓ Now it's doubly important to take care of yourself: A young child needs you to be there for him or her.

✓ Now you have someone else to think of first—a tall order when you have trouble resisting impulses to do what you want right now.

✓ Emotional control is more critical than ever since young kids inevitably try their parents' patience and also haven't developed the executive functions to control themselves.

✓ Kids can't express themselves clearly all the time, meaning it's your job to figure out what they need from you . . . what you should say and when to stay silent . . . when to be firm and when to yield. All of this requires the sophisticated give-and-take skills mentioned above.

Now add in the possibility that your child may also have ADHD.

Research suggests that 30–54% of the children of adults with ADHD will have ADHD.

Obviously having ADHD will make it hard for your child to understand and follow your rules, to remember to do chores and homework, to control emotions when frustrated or tired, and to behave well at home and in public.

Our own study found that the children of adults with ADHD were also more likely to be oppositional and defiant *even if they did not have ADHD.*

 If ADHD is genetic, does that mean I shouldn't have children?

Of course not. ADHD is not a deadly disease or severe developmental disability that could give your children an automatic death sentence or leave them in some lifelong vegetative state. Those are the things that might cause parents to avoid having children if it could be predicted that they would occur. Having ADHD is not a life sentence of distress and failure either. Consider the odds for a moment.

If your own ADHD was not the result of genetics (it doesn't run in your family and your own case may have arisen from prenatal factors such as premature birth), then your child's chances of having ADHD are the same as anyone else's—5 to 7.5%. That is no reason not to have children; if it were, no one would procreate.

Now even if your own adult ADHD is of the genetic type, it doesn't guarantee your child will have ADHD either. Yes, the chances will have gone up. Your offspring have a 20–50% chance of having the disorder. But that also means you have a 50–80% chance of having a child who does *not* have the disorder. When it's put that way, you can see that the chances are pretty decent you may not have a child with ADHD.

Even if your children do have ADHD, it's the most treatable disorder in psychiatry, so it can be managed successfully, especially when identified and treated early. And having ADHD doesn't mean your child cannot have a long, productive, and happy life. When the disorder is managed properly, many children and adults with ADHD wind up having fulfilling lives and contribute to our society in useful and even important ways.

Good Parenting with ADHD

✓ Get your ADHD evaluated and treated. You can't raise your children as well as you would wish to do if your own ADHD is making it hard to control your behavior.

✓ If you see the signs of ADHD in your child, or you have other concerns about the child's psychological development, have him or her evaluated and treated by a qualified mental health professional. Having an undiagnosed and untreated parent with ADHD raising an undiagnosed and untreated child with the disorder is a recipe for chronic conflict and other psychological disasters.

> Guilt, fear, and a desire to avoid more stress may make you downplay signs of ADHD you see in your child. In that case try to trust your spouse or other close relative without ADHD who reports the same concerns.

✓ ADHD can make parents pay less attention to their kids and reward them less. Try to set aside certain times to devote to your child. Use external cues to remind you of these "appointments" and of the rewards you want to give your child for the achievements and behavior all parents want to encourage.

✓ If it is after school, a weekend, summer vacation, or any other time when your children are home or in the yard and you're responsible for

Several studies show that parents with ADHD are less likely to monitor their children's activities than other parents. Lack of monitoring is one of several factors that raise the risk of accidental injuries in those children. This may explain, in part, why children with ADHD have more injuries of all types than other kids—many of their parents have ADHD.

supervising, set an external timer to frequent intervals, such as every 15 to 30 minutes, to remind you to stop what you're doing and monitor your children's activities and whereabouts. This is even more important if your children also have ADHD.

✓ Inconsistency is the bugaboo of parents with ADHD. You might be a harsh taskmaster one day and your child's fairy godmother the next. Or you might just react impulsively to every (mis)behavior with off-the-cuff comments, directives, commands, or reprimands. This is confusing to kids. Talk through the family rules with your child's other parent, write them down, and keep them posted where you'll be reminded of them constantly while at home. Buy yourself time whenever you find yourself confronted by aggravating behavior from your child so you can use the responses you've mutually decided on.

> See Chapter 16 for stop-the-action strategies and Chapter 19 for use of external cues.

✓ Parents with ADHD also seem to be less adept at problem solving when confronted with a child's behavior problems. Use all the arrows in your quiver to learn problem solving. It will model a crucial skill for your child while helping you avoid conflict in the moment.

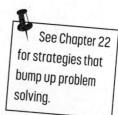

> See Chapter 22 for strategies that bump up problem solving.

✓ Take a behavioral parent training class at a nearby mental health clinic, medical school, university, hospital, or county mental health center. Most large metropolitan areas have such resources. If you live in a rural area lacking such services or can't find a parenting class, consider reading our book *Your Defiant Child* (Guilford Press, 2013) to learn more about methods that can be very helpful in raising a child with ADHD. For teens, see our book *Your Defiant Teen* (Guilford Press, 2013). Parents with ADHD do not do well in these classes if their own ADHD is not being treated, so treat your own ADHD before starting one of these classes. If you live in Canada, you can get online parent training classes, often live, at the Strongest Families website (*strongestfamilies.com*).

✓ Put yourself in time-out (a quiet room) if you're feeling overwhelmed or stressed by your child.

✓ Build in weekly respites from your kids. Find some hobby, club, organization, project, or recreational activity you love that renews you emotionally, de-stresses you, or in other ways gives you time to recharge your parental batteries. Every parent needs some time away every week to regroup, but especially parents with ADHD.

Smart Dual Parenting

These are the types of duties it may be best to delegate to the parent without ADHD:

• *Handling school homework,* especially if your ADHD is untreated. Most parents are not good tutors for their children, so you can bet that this would be true for one with ADHD.

• *Doing all the child care on alternating nights* so that no parent carries the burden of supervising and caring for the children throughout the day or after school. Taking turns like this is especially important when a child has ADHD.

• *Handling time-sensitive events related to the children,* such as medical and school appointments or deadlines for school projects. You can make up for it by taking on tasks that are not time sensitive (like laundry, housecleaning, home and car maintenance, yard care, bathing the children, reading bedtime stories).

• *Driving the kids to their activities whenever possible* (unless you are taking ADHD medication).

• *Approving major child disciplinary actions you want to take* **before** *(!) you implement them.* It's not that you should have no say, but discussing such moves with your partner can prevent poorly thought out and possibly excessive discipline.

Friendships

Do you have a lot of friends? Old friends? Our extensive studies on adults with ADHD revealed significant problems with starting and maintaining social relationships. Adults with ADHD generally say they have fewer close friends than others do, though most said they had some friends. Almost invariably, friendships didn't last as long as for adults without ADHD. Adults with ADHD say they're periodically on the outs with people they consider friends, usually because they couldn't figure out how to resolve normal conflicts or because they couldn't control their anger or other emotions. Sometimes this pattern ends in the adults becoming pretty isolated, even reclusive.

> Research has found that at least 50% and as many as 70% of children with ADHD had no close friends by the time they reached second or third grade. It didn't take weeks or years for other kids to start rejecting those with ADHD but *minutes to hours* after the child with ADHD entered a new peer group, such as children at a summer camp.

Why is this childhood experience relevant to you? Because unless your ADHD has been treated and you've invested effort into using strategies like those in Step Four and developed the social skills usually blocked by ADHD, these difficulties with social relationships have probably followed you into adulthood, just like ADHD has.

What to do about it? Follow all the advice for the other relationships in this chapter. And don't forget the all-important Rule 8 in Step Four: Demonstrate that you can laugh at yourself and that you're trying to overcome the social malaise that ADHD has inflicted. Many friendships are made—and maintained—on a foundation of honesty, humor (self-deprecation), and humility.

28

Driving, Health, and Lifestyle Risks

"It's not just all the speeding and parking tickets I seem to have racked up in my life that explain why I have had my license suspended so many times, though God knows they're enough to explain some of those suspensions. It's also my extreme forgetfulness and this generally bad sense of timing I have. For instance, I neglected to pay a ticket for a citation I got saying my car was 'out of inspection.' The police-man told me that if I forgot to pay it my license would be suspended. So I get that notice, forget to pay it, and now I get arrested for driving on a suspended license. Then I get assigned to traffic school but forget to go on the right date. The problem is that this has happened three times over a single episode of not getting my car inspected. Then I got assigned to go back to traffic school. But I got the date wrong for the starting day, so I miss that class. The judge then orders me to take the next class and to do some community service too. Then I don't follow up with doing the community service the court required, and I am out driving anyway and wind up being charged for driving on a suspended license again. The reason I got stopped and they discovered my license was suspended was—duh!—my car inspection decal was out of date! So this is my fourth time the court has suspended my license for not paying the ticket for an uninspected car!"

"Do I speed with my car? You bet. If I didn't, I couldn't concentrate on the driving part 'cause I'd be fiddling with the radio and changing stations or text messaging one of my friends or doing several things at once without paying much attention to my driving. So, the speeding gets me excited and then I can focus better on the driving itself."

How do you figure out whether something is risky? You look at the conse-quences—that is, *what will happen in the future* as a result.

If you've read this book in order, I'm sure you're way ahead of me here: Without some self-restraint and a good sense of time, how likely are you to be a wise judge of risk?

Not very.

Onlookers in your life may have accused you over the years of indulging in risky behavior. By using the word *indulge* they've been doing you an injustice. *Indulge* implies that you understand the risk and take it anyway. That's not the case.

> If you haven't read this book in order, now is a good time to take a look at Step Two.

Rather, you have deficits in the executive functions that would help you assess risk. To put it simply, where risk is concerned, you usually don't see that there is any.

As a result of this limited foresight and consequent poor risk assessment, plus all the other symptoms of ADHD, you and other adults with the condition have more:

> **ADHD makes you "probability blind"—you don't look ahead to consider seriously and rationally what might happen as a result of whatever actions you're considering taking.**

✓ Driving problems

✓ Accidental injuries

✓ Health problems flowing from reduced concern for health-conscious behavior, which can result in limited exercise, obesity, poor nutrition, impaired sleep, and increased alcohol, tobacco, and marijuana use.

✓ Early pregnancies, early parenthood, and sexually transmitted diseases

Research has documented all of these increased threats to your health, safety, and welfare. Perhaps you've had your share of car accidents and tickets, broken bones and burns, unplanned pregnancies, or regrettable one-night stands, and you'd like to feel and look healthier. It's no wonder that children with ADHD are twice as likely as others to die before age 10 and adults with ADHD over four times more likely to die by age 45, largely due to their risk taking and propensity for accidental injuries. And my own recent research shows that all of these adverse health correlates of having ADHD add up to an average of 11–13 years of reduced life expectancy compared to others of the same age—that's two to six times worse than any of the big health risks public health agencies are so concerned about in adults (smoking, obesity, alcohol use, poor nutrition, lack of exercise). Adult ADHD isn't just a mental health problem; left untreated it's a public health problem too. So, isn't it time to work on avoiding bad risks and stop listening to others ranting about your "indulgences"?

Driving Safely

I'm starting the discussion of risk with driving because problems that occur when an adult with ADHD is behind the wheel are so common—and so potentially deadly.

My research, studies done by others, and even DMV records all show that adults with ADHD are more likely than other adults to have:

✓ Had their driver's license suspended or revoked

✓ Been cited for driving without a valid driver's license

✓ Crashed while driving

✓ Been at fault in such a crash

✓ Had crashes that were two to four times worse in terms of damage and injuries

✓ Been cited for speeding and even reckless driving

Obviously, these are costly consequences. But you may not find them convincing enough to address your own driving problems. That's because, as others have said, "statistics are people with their tears wiped away." So let me tell you a personal story that shows just how costly the driving problems of adults with ADHD can be. Much goes unsaid in this article, not the least of which is that Ron was my twin (fraternal, or nonidentical). Perhaps telling his story will make his tragic loss and that of my family serve some purpose by benefiting you or others you may know with ADHD.

Fatal One-Car Accident in Keene

By Andrea VanValkenburg

Staff Writer, *Press Republican,* Plattsburgh, NY

July 26, 2006

KEENE—An Elizabethtown man died Monday night when his vehicle overturned after hitting an embankment. Ronald Barkley, 56, was traveling southbound on the Bartlett Road in Keene around 10:06 P.M. when he failed to negotiate a small bend in the road and veered off the shoulder of the right lane. According to Ray Brook–based State Police, . . . Barkley was ejected from the GMC Safari minivan during the crash and was pinned underneath as the car overturned. A passerby noticed the accident shortly after it occurred and contacted area officials. Within minutes, State Police and volunteers from the Keene Fire Department responded to the accident, but Barkley was pronounced dead upon arrival. According to police, Barkley was traveling at an unsafe speed when the accident occurred. Investigators believe he was not wearing a seat belt at the time of the accident. An autopsy was conducted at the Adirondack Medical Center Tuesday, which determined Barkley died of head trauma. No further information was available Tuesday night.

My brother Ron had moderate to severe ADHD dating back to early childhood, which continued throughout his life—a life that ended abruptly and violently on a Monday evening in the summer of 2006. That fatal accident was attributable indirectly to his ADHD and more directly to the condition's impact on the driving patterns and habits—speeding, risk taking, distractibility while driving, use of alcohol, and rarely using a seat belt—that conspired to prematurely end his life that fateful evening.

The context of Ron's accident is worth noting. He was simply out for a pleasure drive along a rural dirt road on a fine summer evening, enjoying the beautiful scenery of the Adirondack Mountains as he so often loved to do. He had finished working a 10-hour shift as a chef and had a drink with our 92-year-old mother shortly before grabbing some dinner and then departing on his pleasure drive in a used van he had just bought and proudly fixed up. Perhaps he had also had a few more drinks with his dinner before departing—we can only hazard a guess about that, but his death certificate cited intoxication as a contributing factor in his crash and death. A few days earlier we had spoken by phone, and he was the happiest I had heard him lately, owing to his new job and the fact that, after years of doing various odd jobs and mostly playing guitar and singing in rock bands, he was finally going to get employee benefits.

You see, Ron had quit high school at age 16 after his second attempt at 10th grade, which he was in the midst of failing again. He took up playing the guitar and eventually became extremely proficient in rock and blues music. He would go on to be in countless bands over the next 40 years along the East Coast and in southern California. Clearly he was a gifted musician, and many would listen in awe as he played. And he was the life of the party, always talking, cutting up and making jokes, doing silly things, or just being entertaining. But he had no head for business, a penchant for spending money beyond his means, and no time management skills. He was quick to anger and was generally very impulsive, as well as prone to boredom in whatever job he currently held. So he drifted from band to band and, when not working in music, was likely to be working as a cook in restaurants to help make ends meet. He had two failed marriages and many short-term cohabiting relationships with women. He had a long history of alcohol, tobacco, and, especially, cocaine abuse. He did a few stints in jail for drug possession or sale. He couldn't seem to stay at any job for long. Eventually Ron fathered three children but could never seem to provide the sustained care and support they required, and so wound up with child support payments and often little or no custody of his children.

More to the point here, Ron's driving record was pretty atrocious. Nearly every risk factor identified in research studies—mine and others'—was present in Ron's driving history, and in his tragic accident and consequently untimely demise. It's a powerful irony not lost on me as an expert on both ADHD and its consequences for driving. For recent studies make it abundantly clear that irreparable harm can befall those with ADHD (and others!) during this relatively mundane activity. Just as clear is the fact that those driving problems are responsive to medication treatments—treatments my brother was always too reluctant or distracted to obtain or sustain for very long.

Problems with driving are found to be more frequent in different types of studies looking at both teens and adults, but especially in adults clinically diagnosed with ADHD. Those particular studies find that adults with ADHD, like my brother:

✓ Have slower and more variable reaction times

✓ Make more impulsive errors

✓ Vary in their steering

✓ Are far more inattentive and distractible while driving than other adults

✓ Are less likely to wear a seat belt or to keep their attention on the road instead of fiddling with the stereo controls or radio stations, text messaging or talking on cell phones while driving, or just socializing too much with others in the vehicle

✓ Are more prone to road rage, or driving-related anger and aggressive use of a motor vehicle when angered

These things were all true for my brother.

The most common cause of car accidents is driver inattention. It's therefore easy to see why adults with ADHD are far more likely to:

✓ Have more severe crashes as measured by dollar damages and injuries

✓ Drink alcohol and drive

✓ Be more impaired from that alcohol than others

> Adults with ADHD not only get three to five times as many speeding tickets but also get more parking tickets—impulsively parking wherever they are because they lack the patience to look for a legal spot.

All of these were involved in my brother's deadly accident.

Even more telling than the fact that adults with ADHD have more driving incidents than others is *how much more often* they have them:

✓ An average of *three times more* license suspensions/revocations

> Adults with ADHD are 2.5 times more likely than other adults to die prematurely from misadventures like car accidents.

✓ *Fifty percent more* crashes

✓ Nearly *three times more* speeding tickets

✓ *More than twice as many* accidents in which they were at fault

✓ *More than twice as many* speeding tickets and total citations on their DMV records

Safety Strategies

Fortunately, recent studies have shown that driving performance can be improved by the ADHD medications (stimulants and atomoxetine, although the stimulants appear more effective here). Be diligent about this:

✓ If your ADHD is moderate to severe, be sure you're taking your ADHD medication whenever you drive.

✓ Also take your medication if operating vehicles or heavy equipment is part of your work.

✓ What is also important here is to take your medication on a schedule that ensures you'll have adequate levels of medication in your bloodstream when you're most likely to be driving, such as morning and evening commuting or late-night driving for work or social occasions. Earlier doses, even of extended-release compounds, may wear off too soon; many adults take a "booster" of immediate-release medication later in the day to make sure they're covered. *Your life and the lives of others on the road are at stake.*

✓ If you're not taking medication or there's a chance it has worn off, *let someone else drive.* Forget your pride; let your spouse, friend, or other licensed driver get behind the wheel while you enjoy the scenery and fiddle with the music from the passenger seat.

✓ *Always* (!) wear your seat belt. You can put a sticky note on your dashboard—or, better yet, over the ignition—to remind you to put it on before heading out. I don't want you to wind up like my brother, who was thrown from his van during a minor low-speed rollover and crushed by his own vehicle.

✓ *Absolutely NO alcohol should be consumed when you plan to operate a motor vehicle.* Period.

✓ Stay off your cell phone while driving. This is one of the most frequent sources of distraction while driving, contributing to your crash risk, and you, as an adult with ADHD, do not need more distractions. If you need to use the phone or answer a call, text message, or e-mail, *get off the road!* Then respond. *Never, ever, ever* do it while you're driving. If you simply cannot resist, buy an app that will block your signals or deactivate your phone while the car is turned on and/or moving. Check the app store for your smartphone to see if they have an app that will deactivate your cell phone when it is moving faster than it is possible for a human to walk. For a review of these apps, go to *insuramatch.com/blog/2017/08/apps-prevent-phone-use-while-driving.* These inventions could solve your cell phone or texting dependency and that of other drivers in your family as well.

Studies show that adults with ADHD:

- Already drive as if they are legally intoxicated even if they have had no alcohol
- Are more adversely affected in their driving by even low doses of alcohol than drivers without ADHD

Avoiding Injuries

ADHD can be a life-threatening disorder.

You're not just at risk for car accidents but for all kinds of accidental injuries.

One study found that children with ADHD (and other disruptive behavior problems) were three times more likely to die before the age of 46 than children without these disorders (3% versus 1%).

According to various studies, kids with ADHD are more likely to spend time in a hospital burn unit, to be involved in pedestrian–auto or bicyclist–auto accidents, to be poisoned, to break bones, to have head injuries, and to lose teeth than other kids. If you grew up with ADHD, the emergency room may have come to feel like your home away from home. In fact, the accidents that children with ADHD have tend to be more severe than those that other kids suffer too. And they have more such accidents than others do. No wonder their mothers describe a lot more of them as "accident prone."

What about today? As you may well know, these risks continue into adulthood.

My recent research and studies done by others have found that adults with ADHD are:

- Almost 50% more likely to have experienced a serious injury in their lifetimes

- Four times as likely to have had a serious accidental poisoning

- More likely to file claims for worker's compensation than other adults

What can you do about it?

✓ Counteract your **impulsiveness.** Lack of impulse control may lead you to leap in and act without considering the risk of injury. One patient of mine told me that when he was a child he and his friends pitched in to build a ramp out of snow that they could use to ride their sleds down a hill and then sail across a heavily traveled town road. But when the ramp was finished, he was the only one actually willing to try it. He wound up landing on a car with his sled rather than clearing the road and was seriously injured. Such stories are, unfortunately, more common in the life histories of adults with ADHD than in those without the disorder. Practice the stop-the-action strategies in Chapter 16.

✔ **Take medication to reduce your distractibility and inattentiveness.** Riding your bike on a busy road or crossing the street on foot, you're much less likely than other adults to pay attention to the traffic and avoid potential accidents. **Also practice self-talk and mental imagery** (see Chapters 17 and 18) to help you focus your attention before starting a potentially risky activity and while engaging in it.

✔ While you're practicing self-talk, **ask yourself whether you're being childishly rebellious or grandiose** when you refuse to take conventional safety measures. Sixty-five percent or more of the kids who have ADHD are also defiant. If you were among them as a child, you may have a pretty firmly entrenched habit of ignoring other people's rules and may think you can get away with ignoring a risk.

✔ **Know your physical limits.** Children with ADHD may be more clumsy and less coordinated than others in their motor skills and development. Sometimes adults don't fully catch up. If you know you're not that coordinated, be humble, follow Rule 8 (see Chapter 23), and laugh at yourself—and then put on that bike helmet, buckle your seat belt, or run on the sidewalk, not the street.

Making Sex a Less Risky Business

There are only a few studies on the sexual activities of teens and adults with ADHD, two of which were done by my research team. We found that children with ADHD started having intercourse an average of a year earlier than other kids, had more partners, used contraception less, and ended up with nearly *10 times* more teen pregnancies (as either the father or the mother) and *four times* as many sexually transmitted diseases. By age 27 (6 years later) the same group had become equal to the general population in contraception and sexually transmitted diseases, but those with ADHD were still having kids younger.

> Websites like *advocatesforyouth.org* share information on sexuality for teenagers and young adults.

What do we advise adults with ADHD to do? Well, there is absolutely no research on interventions that may work for these problems, but here are some obvious suggestions to try:

✔ If you left school before finishing sex education classes, get educated. Every major bookstore has a section of books on sex and health. You will even come across "owner's manuals" that tell you how to take care of your body that will contain chapters on sex. Use the Internet. The point here is to inform yourself about sex, contraception, and related topics so you can better manage your sex life.

Several studies by my friend and colleague Eric J. Mash, PhD, and his students at the University of Calgary (Canada) found that pregnant women with ADHD were less likely to be married and less likely to have planned their pregnancies than women without ADHD. The mothers with ADHD were also more likely to be anxious and depressed both before and after their children were born. Before birth the mothers had less positive expectations about motherhood, and after birth they had more difficulty with child rearing.

✓ Unless you are planning on having a child, ALWAYS (!) use contraception. For women, this is easier because of birth control pills that can be taken daily. Both men and women have to remember to carry and use condoms, however, since the pill does not prevent sexually transmitted diseases. Unfortunately, this is just one more thing to be forgotten in the heat of the sexual moment. If you have a history of impulsive sexual activity that you've regretted, get your doctor to prescribe the morning-after pill, which can reduce the risk of conception after the fact. Or consider getting the Norplant subcutaneous form of birth control, which involves having a small device implanted (typically) just below the surface of the skin on your upper arm that emits birth control medication over extended periods of time. If you're older and have had as many children as you want, a vasectomy for men or a tubal ligation for women is an option you can consider to alleviate the need to remember contraception. Still, however, you'll need to take adequate measures to avoid sexually transmitted diseases.

✓ Consider getting the human papillomavirus (HPV) vaccination, which can now be given even to children. On average, people with ADHD have more sex partners across their active sexual life than do other people. Besides a family history of the disease, the single best predictor of cervical, throat, and anal cancer (all of which can be caused by an HPV infection) is the number of sex partners. The HPV vaccination can prevent infection by a virus known to increase the risk for all of these cancers. A vaccine is now available for men as well as women.

Reducing Health and Lifestyle Risks

As an adult with ADHD, you need to pay more attention to common health and lifestyle risks than most adults. ADHD makes you:

✓ More vulnerable to substance use and dependence (see Chapter 30), including the legal substances caffeine, nicotine, and alcohol

✓ More likely to be overweight due to less exercise, more sedentary activities like watching TV or playing video games, and a less healthy diet than other adults

✓ Less likely to have preventive medical and dental care and thus more likely to end up with undetected problems that become bigger problems, such as infected teeth that can cause sepsis or heart infections or obesity, which can cause type 2 diabetes.

These ADHD-related health and lifestyle habits put you at greater risk for coronary artery disease and cancer, among other medical and dental problems.

Again, ADHD can literally be a life-threatening illness. The very nature of ADHD symptoms, particularly those of impaired inhibition and self-control, puts you at risk for a shorter life span. If you can't seriously consider the future consequences of your behavior, you're not going to be nearly concerned enough about health-conscious behavior, such as exercise, proper diet, and moderate use of caffeine, tobacco, and alcohol.

Studies show that half of all deaths in the United States are the result of lifestyle choices in areas such as:

1. Tobacco use (19%)

2. Diet and physical activity (14%)

3. Alcohol use (5%)

4. Firearm use (2%)

5. Sexual behavior (1%)

6. Driving (1%)

7. Illicit drug use (1%)

Canadian research also found that 50% of all premature deaths could have been prevented through lifestyle changes across similar domains.

Then there's conscientiousness, considered one of five major personality dimensions. To be conscientious is to tend toward the *opposite* of ADHD symptoms—to control impulses, think about the consequences of your actions, persist toward goals, and so forth. We now know that conscientiousness is linked to your risk for various health problems and even to your life expectancy.

Because you have ADHD symptoms in place of innate conscientiousness, you're going to need more assistance from medical and health professionals who are expert in the management of these health risks and lifestyle problem areas, in the form of smoking cessation programs, dietary management, exercise regimens, and so forth.

Don't let ADHD shorten your life expectancy because of its association with these risk factors! Take whatever measures you can to (1) control your ADHD and (2) strive for a healthy lifestyle now. ADHD seems to take a higher toll over time.

What can you do to start protecting your health and longevity today?

People diagnosed with ADHD during adulthood were about as active physically as adults in the general population. But adults (age 27) who had had ADHD since childhood and were followed to adulthood were *significantly less likely to get regular routine exercise* (44% versus 69% of the general population). *If this pattern continues, these adults will be more prone to health problems stemming from lack of exercise later in life.*

✓ Make an appointment for a physical with your doctor if it's been a while since you had one or you've never had one as an adult. This is a status check to see what problems or issues are developing and to try to head them off early with better preventive medical care. You avoid medical care at your own long-term risk, so don't play the odds thinking that because you feel well or have no obvious current medical problems some are not festering unseen or undetected. Get a baseline physical and follow the advice your doctor may give you.

✓ If you smoke, ask your doctor to recommend a smoking cessation program to get you to stop.

If you're overweight, ADHD medication can be doubly beneficial to you since it often causes weight loss.

✓ Drinking a lot? It's hard to be the judge of your own behavior, especially if you're in denial. But if someone else tells you the amount you're drinking is excessive, try to listen. Consider making a little check mark on a small piece of

> **Uninsured and can't afford to see a doctor?**
>
> - See if a parent, sibling, or other relative would cover this cost for you.
> - Check with the local county or city hospital about getting a physical at the county's or state's expense if you fall below the poverty line in your income.
> - Call your local department of social services to see if they can direct you to free care clinics.

paper every time you have a drink and then look at the pattern over a week. Is it more than you used to drink? Is it more than your family and friends drink? Do you get hangovers often or just feel slow and sluggish in the mornings after drinking? Talk to your doctor, who is there to help, not judge. If you have a problem, ask your doctor to enroll you in a nearby alcohol rehabilitation program and Alcoholics Anonymous (AA) group or another ongoing support program for recovering alcoholics.

✓ Ditto with drugs. Your doctor can help you enroll in a drug detox clinic or other local program.

✓ Be sure to see a dentist. Dental problems or diseases left unchecked could cause you to lose some or all of your teeth, require a partial or full set of dentures, or lead to more extensive dental or gum surgery, or possibly even abscessed teeth, which have the potential to be lethal if that infection happens to enter your bloodstream and attack your heart.

✓ Start a plan of regular physical exercise each week. All of us struggle with this sound advice, but that's no excuse for any of us not to try to make this a more routine part of our lifestyle. There is also the added benefit that physical exercise done regularly helps people with ADHD manage their symptoms better and provides a great release for all that extra energy and hyperactivity. My patients and other adults with ADHD tell me that running, biking, swimming, other aerobic sports, and even martial arts, have proven helpful to them in reducing their symptoms by channeling their energy into a healthier outlet.

✓ Consider medication to treat your ADHD. Often the medical and dental risks identified in our research on adults with ADHD stem from unmanaged ADHD and the disorganizing effects it has on their life. Getting your ADHD under control with medication can help you pursue preventive medicine and dentistry as required for all adults.

29

Other Mental and Emotional Problems

If you've been struggling for years with the symptoms of ADHD without knowing what's wrong, being diagnosed can be a huge relief. Not only do you finally have an explanation for your problems. You also have access to proven treatments that can alleviate your symptoms and put success within your reach.

But what if medications and the self-help strategies described in this book aren't enough? What do you do if your days still seem awfully hard to get through? If you still can't get ahead at work, finish your education, enjoy your family and social life? If you still feel miserable and frustrated much of the time, what could be going on?

Consider the possibility that ADHD is not the only mental or emotional condition you have. In Chapter 1, I said that 80% or more of adults with ADHD have at least one other psychiatric disorder. More than 50% have at least two other disorders. These are the most common culprits, listed roughly from most to least prevalent:

> Having another disorder besides ADHD doesn't make you unusual or beyond help. Only 1 in 5 adults with ADHD has ADHD alone.

✓ Oppositional defiant disorder (ODD)

✓ Conduct disorder (CD)/antisocial personality disorder (ASPD)

✓ Substance use disorders

✓ Anxiety

✓ Depression

✓ Personality disorders (such as antisocial or borderline personality disorder)

✓ Binge-eating disorder or bulimia (in women)

✓ Learning disabilities

The rates at which these conditions have been found in adults with ADHD vary from study to study, so this order is not set in stone. But it will give you an idea of what might be ailing you when ADHD doesn't explain all the obstacles in the way of your having the life you want.

In the following pages I'll give you a basic understanding of what some of these conditions look (and feel) like and also how they are usually treated by a mental health professional. Of course the only way to be sure that you have any of these disorders is to get a thorough evaluation and diagnosis.

If you've already been diagnosed with ADHD, why wouldn't the evaluator have noticed anything else that was wrong too? In an ideal world, your evaluation for ADHD *would* have uncovered any other conditions you have. But on this imperfect planet, a lot of factors could have kept other conditions from revealing themselves. Maybe you and the evaluator were so fixed on the idea of ADHD that you downplayed other symptoms that lurked in the background of your history. Maybe these other conditions were so mild at the time that they really didn't qualify for a diagnosis. It's always possible that the diagnosing practitioner was inexperienced—in general or in identifying psychiatric disorders other than ADHD. It could even be that your doctor saw the signs of other problems but believed it would be best to have you focus on ADHD and get that under control before being asked both to accept that you have other conditions on top of it and to participate in managing them.

Call your doctor, ideally the same one who diagnosed you with ADHD, and ask for a consultation. Be prepared to describe the symptoms you're experiencing, the impairments that seem to be "left over" from your ADHD treatment, and the areas of life in which you're struggling. The following will help you help the practitioner by zeroing in on what's wrong.

Do you often feel mad at the world? _____

_____

Is losing your temper a regular, probably daily, occurrence? _____

_____

Do you think people view you as a maverick, a rule breaker, a rebel? _____

_____

Do you tend to defend yourself relentlessly when someone says you've done something wrong? _____

_____

Have many of the jobs you've left ended because you were fired?

_____

_____

Oppositional Defiant Disorder

The more "yes" answers you gave, the more likely it is that you could have ODD. If what's making you miserable, despite an improvement in your ADHD symptoms thanks to medication, is feeling like a misfit, always the "bad boy," misunderstood and disliked, hemmed in and pushed around, ODD may be the cause. If you remember feeling hostile and stubborn as a child, behaving in ways that adults defined as defiant and that always seemed to get you in trouble, you could have had ODD then even if it wasn't diagnosed. *Among kids who did have these symptoms, the disorder persists into adulthood in fully half.* What causes it? We're not sure. It could be the limited emotional self-control that is inherent in ADHD, and being constantly at odds with adults trying to make them behave in ways they can't because of their deficits in executive function. By the time kids have had ADHD symptoms for 2 or 3 years, *45–84% of them have ODD too.* But it also could be that the emotion regulation problems presented by ADHD create a major predisposition to problems with managing anger and frustration. Certainly, the impulsive emotion associated with ADHD leads to a greater quickness to anger, impatience, and low frustration tolerance, which can be the initial spark for the fires of ODD. Venting and acting out with others leads to lots of conflict, especially with authority figures. Maybe that's why adults with ODD are more likely to get fired, even though poor work performance ratings are more often traceable to ADHD.

Treatment: In many cases, the medication used to treat ADHD also improves ODD. By facilitating emotional control and other types of self-control that help you fit into society more comfortably, the medication you're already taking may diminish the ODD symptoms over time. If the ADHD medications have not completely managed your impulsive emotions, consider enrolling in an anger management course with a mental health professional, nearby mental health clinic, or community college. Or try the self-help methods in W. Robert Nay's *Taking Charge of Anger* (Guilford Press, 2012). Also, some adults require a second medication just to manage this aspect of their problems beyond the medications traditionally used to treat ADHD. Ask your doctor about them.

Did you get in trouble with the law as a child or teen? _____

Run away from home? _____

Get caught for truancy or curfew violations? _____

How about now? Do you have a criminal record? _____

Do you push the envelope on laws, community ordinances, rules and regulations? _____

Have you been kicked out of the house? _____

Have a history of alcohol and/or drug abuse? _____

Do you get involved in bar fights? _____

Have you ever been accused of sexual harassment or assault?

_____

Conduct Disorder/Antisocial Personality Disorder

Many who answered "yes" to a lot of the questions above wouldn't even be reading this book. But to those who are: If you have a history of criminal or near-criminal behavior, you may still be struggling despite treating your ADHD because you've become somewhat marginalized in society. It could take time and professional counseling to get you back into the mainstream.

You could think of CD as a step up (or down) from ODD. Kids and teens who have CD aren't just defiant. They lie, steal, fight, carry weapons, set fires, and/or commit sexual assault—generally violating the rights of others and social norms and laws. While the great majority of adults with ADHD don't qualify for this diagnosis, 17–35% can remember fitting this profile closely enough to have qualified for the diagnosis when younger. Those who still fit this picture as adults—anywhere from 7 to 21% of those who still have ADHD (with my own follow-up study revealing the higher number)—would be diagnosed currently with ASPD, which is essentially CD grown up. How does someone develop such severe behavior problems? Partly as a result of the problems with inhibition and self-regulation that go with ADHD. But those symptoms can't explain everything, since most people with ADHD don't end up with CD or ASPD too. More likely, it's ADHD *combined* with other factors including genetic risks for CD, drug-abuse-related disorders in the parents, a disruptive home life, social disadvantage, being raised by a single parent, reduced parental monitoring of a teen's activities, and affiliation with delinquent or drug-using peers in adolescence. As noted in Chapter 30, drug abuse and antisocial behavior seem to go hand in hand.

> Substance use disorders affect a significant minority of adults with ADHD. They are addressed separately in Chapter 30.

Treatment: See the treatment options listed for ODD. Also, get help for substance use if you have a problem there. And always remember that antisocial friends are no friends at all. Do what you can to exit a social scene that encourages crime and other antisocial behavior. Keep busy with hobbies if you must. Ideally, though, identify a better social network that encourages positive, productive activity. If necessary, move to a different neighborhood with fewer antisocial peers to interact with on a frequent basis.

Does anticipating things you don't want to do make you extremely nervous? _____

Do you worry about a laundry list of possible events all the time?

_____

Do you have any phobias (as in extreme fear of spiders, heights)?

_____

Do social occasions fill you with fear, often making you cancel at the last minute? _____

Do you hate speaking before a group? _____

Anxiety

Anxiety can be hard to recognize. It's usually defined as a pattern of abnormal fears and worries, mainly unrealistic ones, often about things that will never occur. In your case, though, it may seem perfectly reasonable to avoid entering the same social situation in which you've been humiliated dozens of times before. Or it's entirely logical to quake in fear before addressing a meeting at work when the other times you've lost your place, forgotten your materials, or frozen during the question-and-answer period. Isn't it sensible to protect yourself from disasters that actually *have* occurred before? It may very well be, but that doesn't mean that you're not suffering from clinical anxiety that could be treated, making your life a whole lot easier. About a quarter of the kids with ADHD have an anxiety disorder, but among adults the rate climbs to 17–52%. In our follow-up study of children with ADHD in Wisconsin, my colleague Mariellen Fischer and I found that the longer you have ADHD as an adult, the more likely it is that you'll develop an anxiety disorder too. I think it makes sense to assume that a history of chronic failure in various domains of major life activity could be to blame. But there may also be some shared genetic risk between the two disorders. Watch for new findings in the research news.

Treatment: There are many psychotherapy treatments for anxiety, especially cognitive-behavioral therapy, as well as drugs proven to help. Remember that the ADHD nonstimulant atomoxetine may be of some benefit since it does not exacerbate anxiety and may treat it to some extent. Ask your doctor what's best for you.

Do you often find it hard to get out of bed and feel exhausted even after plenty of sleep? _____

Do you feel blue more days than not? _____

Do you snap at people, feeling easily irritated? _____

Is your appetite dead . . . or in overdrive? _____

Do you feel bored with and uninterested in activities you usually enjoy?

_____

Depression

"Yes" answers to many of those questions are clues that you may be suffering from depression. But the research on the risk of depression among adults with ADHD is rather mixed. So we can't say that you should be on the lookout for these symptoms because you're strongly predisposed to become depressed at some point. Overall, the risk for some type of depression is more than three times greater in people with ADHD than in the general population samples we've used as control groups. Interestingly, unlike anxiety, my Wisconsin follow-up study showed that depression dropped from 28% in childhood to 18% by age 27. Research shows that there may be a shared genetic risk between the two disorders. That is, having one disorder in your family seems to predispose you to having biological relatives with the other. But the environment could be to blame too. Both depression and ADHD are associated with a greater exposure to social turmoil, stress, disadvantage, and abuse.

Treatment: As for anxiety, there are many effective medications for depression (antidepressants), as well as proven cognitive-behavioral approaches.

> A few studies have suggested that adults with ADHD might be more at risk for bipolar disorder (manic depression), but *most studies,* including my own, have not found this to be the case. Adults with bipolar disorder *do,* however, have a higher risk for ADHD. That risk is 20–25% for adult-onset bipolar disorder, 35–45% for adolescent onset, and 80–97% if the bipolar disorder started in childhood.

30

Drugs and Crime

"When I was a teenager, and even into my 20s, I was hanging around with a few guys who, like me, were looking for thrills on weekend nights. So we went barhopping and did a lot of drinking and often just waited for someone else in the bar to say something we didn't like or thought was stupid and we would start a fight with them. I got into so many fights, I can't remember how many. We got thrown out of a lot of bars for doing this, and we often had some injuries from it, but that didn't stop us from going out again the next weekend. Maybe we were just bored or trying to show off for the women in the bars, but for whatever reason, the drinking just made us more brave and also more impulsive and we just did stupid things as a result.

"Once we left a bar after lots of beers and saw a car in the lot with the keys left in it. One of my friends said, 'Hey, let's go for a joy ride!' So we did. We were all liquored up and daring each other to drive the car faster, take it into fields or golf courses and spin doughnut rings, and just tear ass around neighborhoods until we wrecked the car and got arrested for grand theft auto. Boy, we were young, dumb, drunk, and stupid in those days. And my impulsiveness just got worse when I drank. I'm surprised I'm still alive to talk about it.

"But one day I met a guy from high school who I knew and who just always seemed to have his act together and be on the right course. He talked me into trying an alcohol detox clinic where he volunteered to work as a crisis counselor. When I got cleaned up from the booze, I tried out and passed the fireman's exam and became a local volunteer firefighter after my initial training for it. That eventually led me to a paid job with the town as a firefighter. And then I met Karen, who's now my wife, and she really cleaned up my life and gave me a great reason to live, be straight, stay off the booze, get my ADHD diagnosed and treated, and keep my life together. All those guys I used to hang out and barhop with are now in jail. I am the only one who made something of my life."

There is no question that adults with ADHD are more likely to use various substances than other adults. Alcohol is the most frequently abused substance—up to a third of adults with ADHD have or have had a drinking problem. But marijuana, cocaine or other stimulants, prescription drugs, and opiates (heroin, morphine, opium) are also abused, though at a slightly lower rate.

. . . .

Use of cocaine and other hard drugs and abuse of prescription drugs are associated more with CD or other antisocial behavior (see Chapter 29) than ADHD.

. . . .

The trouble is that the nature of substance use disorders, combined with the nature of ADHD, can make it awfully difficult to see yourself as having a "real" problem. People in the general population often take a long time to recognize that they need help and then seek it. With self-awareness limited by the executive function deficits of ADHD, admitting that you have and then addressing a substance use disorder can be even harder.

If you're starting to wonder whether you feel bad despite ADHD treatment because you might qualify for a diagnosis of drug dependence or abuse, this chapter will help you decide what to do.

What Are You Getting Out of Substance Use?

Giving up a substance we enjoy—especially one that we've come to believe we *need*—is hardly a pleasant prospect. Most experts agree that people are often at least trying to get some positive effect from the substances they overuse or abuse. For many of us, alcohol relaxes us and lowers our inhibitions, often making it easier to be sociable and alleviating shyness. But for someone with ADHD and already low inhibition, that could be a social disaster. Nicotine and caffeine stimulate us when we're tired and need to focus. But these typical effects don't completely explain why adults with ADHD are likely to use substances more often than others—to the detriment of their health and well-being. Maybe knowing what you're getting out of the substances that are starting to be a problem for you will help you turn a corner that will preserve your health—or even save your life. Let's look at alcohol first.

Alcohol

Alcohol does not treat the symptoms of ADHD. In fact, it could make them worse. After just a drink or two, alcohol lowers your inhibition, which means it probably gets you into even more trouble than you already have with your impulses.

> **Do you make your worst impulsive decisions after drinking? Such as?**
>
> _____
>
> _____

So what could make you keep drinking? Impulsiveness itself is certainly a candidate. If much of your social life takes place at bars and other places where drinks are served, it just might be hard to resist joining in.

> **Is drinking typically at the center of your get-togethers with friends?**
>
> _____
>
> _____

Much earlier in this book I said you had a lot of options for shaping your environment to manage your ADHD and take charge of your life so ADHD doesn't take charge of you. Your friends are certainly a big part of your environment. Are they the right companions for you?

> **Do you feel like drinking clears your mind of things you don't want to think about?**
>
> _____
>
> _____

After those first few drinks, alcohol is known to restrict one's memory for past events, creating a sort of tunnel vision that focuses awareness mainly on the moment, so you can ignore your past problems. Perhaps that's what makes it so appealing to many adults with ADHD: It helps you forget your troubles and just live in the moment without a care for recent problems or future hazards.

Alcohol is also known to reduce anxiety in some adults. If those things you don't want to think about make you anxious, alcohol may just ease your fears. At least temporarily.

Marijuana

Like alcohol, marijuana is consumed in much greater quantities over the lifetime of adults with ADHD than other adults. Why? That's not clear to me. One possibility is that marijuana may be achieving a similar effect to that of alcohol: helping people with ADHD forget their miseries, focusing their mind just on the moment, and perhaps reducing any unusual levels of anxiety. We do know that those with a history of cigarette smoking are most likely to move on to using marijuana as well. And we know that adults with ADHD are more likely to smoke cigarettes than other adults . . . which leads to one of the most interesting findings about ADHD and substance use:

Cigarettes/Nicotine

Scott Kollins, PhD, and colleagues at Duke University published a 2019 study that shows a direct connection between ADHD and risk for smoking cigarettes. Following 15,197 adolescents into young adulthood, they found a linear relationship between the level of ADHD symptoms and regular smoking. *Specifically, the risk of regular smoking increased significantly with every additional ADHD symptom.* Not only that, but the more ADHD symptoms the teens had, the earlier they started smoking.

Most people wouldn't consider smoking a drug use disorder, but I think it deserves to be viewed this way for a couple of reasons. For one thing, nicotine may very well be the most addictive substance on the planet. For another, we know that smoking comes with some of the deadliest health consequences of any habit we humans have invented (such as lung and other cancers, heart disease). Dependence on or abuse of nicotine is exceptionally common among a sizable minority of adults with ADHD, with their risk for current nicotine use being nearly twice that of the general population. What makes it so seductive?

Some scientists have suggested that this risk for smoking is a form of self-medication. Nicotine has a stimulant-like action on the dopamine transporter in the striatum of the brain that's very similar to the effects of methylphenidate (see Step Three) on that site. **Smoking may actually treat the symptoms of ADHD**

> Caffeine is also considered a stimulant. Not surprisingly, we found that young adults with ADHD in particular were likely to consume more caffeinated drinks per week than young adults without ADHD.

to some degree. Here's a case, though, where the risk (say, of cancer and heart disease) far outweighs the benefits, especially considering that we have safe, legal prescription stimulants to provide the same positive effect.

 I took Ritalin for a long time as a kid. Some people have told me that's probably why I've developed a cocaine habit. Is that true?

Some adults may wonder if having been treated for their ADHD with prescription stimulants as children may have predisposed them toward greater drug use and abuse as adults, especially involving illegal stimulants, or the illegal use of prescription stimulants. I've reviewed the literature on whether treatment with prescription stimulants leads to abuse of stimulants like nicotine, cocaine, crack, or methamphetamine. I can reassure you that at least 16 studies have found no such association between childhood stimulant treatment and adult drug use or abuse. While one study did so, its results were not properly analyzed and so probably yielded a false positive relationship between childhood stimulant use and adult drug use. So the overwhelming majority of the evidence is against such a risk. A few studies, including my own research, showed that being treated with stimulants for ADHD in childhood may actually have protected a child or teen from engaging in certain types of drug use as a young adult, provided that treatment was sustained during adolescence. The effect was a pretty weak one, however, and has not been found consistently across studies. So it's not clear that early treatment can reduce drug abuse risk. But what is pretty definitive is that early treatment with ADHD medications does *not* contribute to a greater risk of drug abuse later in life.

Read on to find out more about why you might be using cocaine.

Cocaine and Other Hard Drugs

Use of illegal drugs like cocaine and "meth" or abuse of legal prescription medications could very well be an attempt to self-medicate ADHD, as with nicotine, since some illegal drugs are stimulants. Talk about a wrong-headed decision!

These drugs, and all the negative consequences of addiction to them, are literally killers.

Why would you choose a dangerous illegal substance instead of a safe legal one? As mentioned earlier, use of cocaine and other hard drugs is associated more with CD, crime, and ASPD (see Chapter 29) than with ADHD. Research clearly shows that teens and young adults with ADHD who are likely to use substances excessively, or who are using or abusing illegal substances, are also the most likely to engage in various antisocial or criminal activities. And substance abuse and criminal activity have a synergistic effect—more crime results in greater drug use, which in turn contributes to yet more crime.

> • • • • • •
> **Antisocial behavior predisposes you to substance use, and substance use predisposes you to antisocial behavior.**
> • • • • • •

Let's say you have a crack habit. How are you going to buy these expensive drugs? You may turn to stealing money or property to obtain the means to buy your drugs of abuse. If you drink alcohol excessively, you may be more likely to get into fights with others. And in both cases, you may be more inclined than others to carry and even use weapons. Similarly, if you engage in certain criminal activities, such as stealing or fighting, you may be doing so with others also prone to antisocial behavior. And those people are more likely to be using drugs and may influence you to do so.

Another link between drug use and antisocial, criminal behavior is impulsivity. The more impulsive you are, studies show, the more likely you are to try an illegal drug on a dare or even a mere suggestion. The same appears to be true of the likelihood of engaging in illegal activities (crime): The more impulsive you are—the less likely you are to consider the consequences of your actions—the more likely it is that you'll yield to a whim or a dare to go along on some criminal misadventure like breaking into a house.

Then we have the kind of social group you hang around with in your spare time. As with drinking, if you pal around with people who are likely to be involved in illegal activities, they may influence you to do the same. Gangs are the most extreme example of this kind of negative social influence, but it doesn't take an organized group like that to exert an influence, especially with ADHD to egg you on. All you may need is a couple of antisocial, drug-using friends to be pushed in this direction.

Our research found that yet another contributor to the risk for engaging in criminal activities is a person's level of education. People with ADHD who had less education, especially if they did not graduate from high school, were far more likely to be doing antisocial things than people with ADHD who graduated or went on after high school to further their education.

Finally, there's the severity of the ADHD and its persistence from childhood

> The type of crime most associated with ADHD in my research was using, possessing, and selling illegal drugs and stealing money to buy drugs. About one in four people with ADHD, at a minimum, are likely to have drug use and abuse issues as adults.
>
> Are you sure you want to be among them?

to adolescence. These factors had a lesser effect but were still important predictors of certain types of criminal behavior in adulthood.

Avoiding—or Getting Out of—the Trap of Drug Use

✓ For the substantial minority of adults with ADHD who have substance use problems (20–30%), drug detoxification and rehabilitation programs are likely to be recommended. It's difficult to treat your ADHD when you're abusing drugs that can make your ADHD worse or lead to other psychological problems in their own right. If you're not getting much benefit from attempts to treat your ADHD, consider whether you need to tackle a substance use problem first or at least simultaneously.

✓ Aggressive treatment of the ADHD is still critical, no matter when you start it.

✓ Change your environment if it's leading you into activities that are making your life worse. Look for new friends (this is one reason 12-step programs like AA are so attractive—they provide a new social arena for those trying to start a new, substance-free phase of their lives). Choose leisure activities that don't center on bars.

✓ Get educated. If your education was cut short by ADHD, get back to it now. A better education means better job opportunities, which can mean not only better opportunities to make a living legally but also removing yourself from living every day on the margins of society.

Substance use and criminal activity—no matter how minor—are major pitfalls for those with adult ADHD. Steer away from them now and start leading the life you deserve.

APPENDIX

A Closer Look at ADHD Symptoms

Official Diagnostic Criteria for ADHD

The official diagnostic criteria used by mental health professionals to diagnose ADHD come from the fifth edition of the *Diagnostic and Statistical Manual of Mental Disorders*, or DSM-5. Practitioners question patients (including adults, although the criteria were developed for use with children) about the 18 symptoms listed below. Nine of these refer to problems with inattention and nine to problems with being hyperactive or impulsive.

DSM-5 Criteria for Attention-Deficit/Hyperactivity Disorder (ADHD)

A. A persistent pattern of inattention and/or hyperactivity–impulsivity that interferes with functioning or development, as characterized by (1) and/or (2):

1. **Inattention:** Six (or more) of the following symptoms have persisted for at least 6 months to a degree that is inconsistent with developmental level and that negatively impacts directly on social and academic/occupational activities:

   Note: The symptoms are not solely a manifestation of oppositional behavior, defiance, hostility, or failure to understand tasks or instructions. For older adolescents and adults (age 17 and older), at least five symptoms are required.

   a. Often fails to give close attention to details or makes careless mistakes in schoolwork, at work, or during other activities (e.g., overlooks or misses details, work is inaccurate).

   b. Often has difficulty sustaining attention in tasks or play activities (e.g., has difficulty remaining focused during lectures, conversations, or lengthy reading).

   c. Often does not seem to listen when spoken to directly (e.g., mind seems elsewhere, even in the absence of any obvious distraction).

    d. Often does not follow through on instructions and fails to finish schoolwork, chores, or duties in the workplace (e.g., starts tasks but quickly loses focus and is easily sidetracked).

    e. Often has difficulty organizing tasks and activities (e.g., difficulty managing sequential tasks; difficulty keeping materials and belongings in order; messy, disorganized work; has poor time management; fails to meet deadlines).

    f. Often avoids, dislikes, or is reluctant to engage in tasks that require sustained mental effort (e.g., schoolwork or homework; for older adolescents and adults, preparing records, completing forms, reviewing lengthy papers).

    g. Often loses things necessary for tasks or activities (e.g., school materials, pencils, books, tools, wallets, keys, paperwork, eyeglasses, mobile telephones).

    h. Is often easily distracted by extraneous stimuli (for older adolescents and adults, may include unrelated thoughts).

    i. Is often forgetful in daily activities (e.g., doing chores, running errands; for older adolescents and adults, returning calls, paying bills, keeping appointments).

2. **Hyperactivity and impulsivity:** Six (or more) of the following symptoms have persisted for at least 6 months to a degree that is inconsistent with developmental level and that negatively impacts directly on social and academic/occupational activities:

    Note: The symptoms are not solely a manifestation of oppositional behavior, defiance, hostility, or a failure to understand tasks or instructions. For older adolescents and adults (age 17 and older), at least five symptoms are required.

    a. Often fidgets with or taps hands or feet or squirms in seat.

    b. Often leaves seat in situations when remaining seated is expected (e.g., leaves his or her place in the classroom, in the office or other workplace, or in other situations that require remaining in place).

    c. Often runs about or climbs in situations where it is inappropriate. (**Note:** In adolescents or adults, may be limited to feeling restless.)

    d. Often unable to play or engage in leisure activities quietly.

    e. Is often "on the go," acting as if "driven by a motor" (e.g., is unable to be or uncomfortable being still for extended time, as in restaurants, meetings; may be experienced by others as being restless or difficult to keep up with).

    f. Often talks excessively.

    g. Often blurts out an answer before a question has been completed (e.g., completes people's sentences; cannot wait for turn in conversation).

    h. Often has difficulty waiting his or her turn (e.g., while waiting in line).

    i. Often interrupts or intrudes on others (e.g., butts into conversations, games, or activities; may start using other people's things without asking or receiving permission; for adolescents and adults, may intrude into or take over what others are doing).

B. Several inattentive or hyperactive–impulsive symptoms were present prior to age 12 years.

C. Several inattentive or hyperactive–impulsive symptoms are present in two or more settings (e.g., at home, school, or work; with friends or relatives; in other activities).

D. There is clear evidence that the symptoms interfere with, or reduce the quality of social, academic, or occupational functioning.

E. The symptoms do not occur exclusively during the course of schizophrenia or another psychotic disorder and are not better explained by another mental disorder (e.g., mood disorder, anxiety disorder, dissociative disorder, personality disorder, substance intoxication or withdrawal).

Specify whether:

314.01 (F90.2) Combined presentation: If both Criterion A1 (inattention) and Criterion A2 (hyperactivity–impulsivity) are met for the past 6 months.

314.00 (F90.0) Predominantly inattentive presentation: If Criterion A1 (inattention) is met but Criterion A2 (hyperactivity–impulsivity) is not met for the past 6 months.

314.01 (F90.1) Predominantly hyperactive/impulsive presentation: If Criterion A2 (hyperactivity–impulsivity) is met and Criterion A1 (inattention) is not met for the past 6 months.

Specify if:

In partial remission: When full criteria were previously met, fewer than the full criteria have been met for the past 6 months, and the symptoms still result in impairment in social, academic, or occupational functioning.

Specify current severity:

Mild: Few, if any, symptoms in excess of those required to make the diagnosis are present, and symptoms result in no more than minor impairments in social or occupational functioning.

Moderate: Symptoms or functional impairment between "mild" and "severe" are present.

Severe: Many symptoms in excess of those required to make the diagnosis, or several symptoms that are particularly severe, are present, or the symptoms result in marked impairment in social or occupational functioning.

The word *often* appears at the beginning of each symptom to ensure that these symptoms are occurring most of the time and are present more often than is the case in other people of your age group. It is also important that these symptoms have been present for at least 6 months to ensure that these are not simply transient problems but are a stable part of your recent life.

Additional Symptoms Associated with ADHD in Adults

To get a better idea of whether you fit the picture of adult ADHD, see how many of the symptoms on pages 272–276 represent your experiences.

Symptom	Adults with ADHD (%)	Adults in the community (%)
1. Find it difficult to tolerate waiting; impatient	75	5
2. Make decisions impulsively	79	3
3. Unable to inhibit my reactions or responses to events or others	61	2
4. Have difficulty stopping my activities or behavior when I should do so	72	2
5. Have difficulty changing my behavior when I am given feedback about my mistakes	68	4
6. Easily distracted by irrelevant thoughts when I must concentrate on something	96	3
7. Prone to daydreaming when I should be concentrating on something	89	8
8. Procrastinate or put off doing things until the last minute	94	27
9. Make impulsive comments to others	56	3
10. Likely to take shortcuts in my work and not do all that I am supposed to do	65	6
11. Likely to skip out on work early if its boring or hard to do	58	5
12. Can't seem to defer gratification or to put off doing things that are rewarding now so as to work for a later goal	69	2
13. Likely to do things without considering the consequences for doing them	60	1
14. Change my plans at the last minute on a whim or last-minute impulse	72	9
15. Start a project or task without reading or listening to directions carefully	89	11
16. Poor sense of time	63	3
17. Waste or mismanage my time	86	5

Note. Results are from *ADHD in Adults: What the Science Says* by Russell A. Barkley, Kevin R. Murphy, and Mariellen Fischer (Guilford Press, 2008).

Symptom	Adults with ADHD (%)	Adults in the community (%)
18. Fail to consider past relevant events or past personal experiences before responding to situations	44	1
19. Do not think about the future as much as others of my age seem to do	47	8
20. Not prepared for work or assigned tasks	58	1
21. Fail to meet deadlines for assignments	65	1
22. Have trouble planning ahead or preparing for upcoming events	81	6
23. Forget to do things I am supposed to do	82	5
24. Have difficulties with mental arithmetic	55	14
25. Not able to comprehend what I read as well as I should be able to do; have to reread material to get its meaning	81	12
26. Can't seem to remember what I previously heard or read about	77	12
27. Can't seem to accomplish the goals I set for myself	84	7
28. Late for work or scheduled appointments	55	5
29. Trouble organizing my thoughts or thinking clearly	75	2
30. Not aware of things I say or do	39	1
31. Can't seem to hold in mind things I need to remember to do	83	7
32. Have difficulty being objective about things that affect me	64	5
33. Find it hard to take other people's perspectives about a problem or situation	48	6
34. Have difficulty keeping in mind the purpose or goal of my activities	51	1
35. Forget the point I was trying to make when talking to others	75	2

Symptom	Adults with ADHD (%)	Adults in the community (%)
36. When shown something complicated to do, cannot keep the information in mind so as to imitate or do it correctly	53	1
37. Give poor attention to details in my work	60	1
38. Find it difficult to keep track of several activities at once	68	8
39. Can't seem to get things done unless there is an immediate deadline	89	6
40. Dislike work or school activities where I must think more than usual	60	2
41. Have difficulty judging how much time it will take to do something or get somewhere	72	6
42. Have trouble motivating myself to start work	80	6
43. Quick to get angry or become upset	63	7
44. Easily frustrated	86	8
45. Overreact emotionally	68	6
46. Have difficulty motivating myself to stick with my work and get it done	84	4
47. Can't seem to persist at things I do not find interesting	96	13
48. Do not put as much effort into my work as I should or as others are able to do	60	4
49. Have trouble staying alert or awake in boring situations	86	11
50. Easily excited by activities going on around me	70	15
51. Not motivated to prepare in advance for things I know I am supposed to do	80	4
52. Can't seem to sustain my concentration on reading, paperwork, lectures, or work	91	7
53. Easily bored	81	9
54. Others tell me I am lazy or unmotivated	57	2
55. Have to depend on others to help me get my work done	44	2

Symptom	Adults with ADHD (%)	Adults in the community (%)
56. Things must have an immediate payoff for me or I do not seem to get them done	70	2
57. Have trouble completing one activity before starting a new one	87	7
58. Have difficulty resisting the urge to do something fun or more interesting when I am supposed to be working	87	5
59. Can't seem to sustain friendships or close relationships as long as other people	46	5
60. Inconsistent in the quality or quantity of my work performance	70	2
61. Don't seem to worry about future events as much as others	46	10
62. Don't think about or talk things over with myself before doing something	48	4
63. Unable to work as well as others without supervision or frequent instruction	40	2
64. Have trouble doing what I tell myself to do	81	5
65. Poor follow-through on promises or commitments I may make to others	68	3
66. Lack self-discipline	81	5
67. Have difficulty using sound judgment in problem situations or when under stress	51	1
68. Trouble following the rules in a situation	61	4
69. Not very flexible in my behavior or approach to a situation; overly rigid in how I like things done	53	16
70. Have trouble organizing my thoughts	80	4
71. Have difficulties saying what I want to say	70	6
72. Unable to come up with or invent as many solutions to problems as others seem to do	37	5
73. Often at a loss for words when I want to explain something to others	58	5
74. Have trouble putting my thoughts down in writing as well or as quickly as others	58	6

Symptom	Adults with ADHD (%)	Adults in the community (%)
75. Feel I am not as creative or inventive as others of my level of intelligence	27	13
76. In trying to accomplish goals or assignments, find I am not able to think of as many ways of doing things as others	41	5
77. Have trouble learning new or complex activities as well as others	56	4
78. Have difficulty explaining things in their proper order or sequence	67	1
79. Can't seem to get to the point of my explanations as quickly as others	75	9
80. Have trouble doing things in their proper order or sequence	76	3
81. Unable to "think on my feet" or respond as effectively as others to unexpected events	37	3
82. Clumsy; not as coordinated in my movements as others	30	6
83. Poor or sloppy handwriting	63	21
84. Have difficulty arranging or doing my work by its priority or importance; can't "prioritize" well	84	4
85. Slower to react to unexpected events	37	5
86. Get silly, clown around, or act foolishly when I should be serious	58	4
87. Can't seem to remember things I have done or places I have been as well as others seem to do	62	14
88. Accident prone	35	3
89. More likely to drive a motor vehicle much faster than others (excessive speeding)	67	13
90. Have difficulties managing my money or credit cards	73	8
91. I am less able to recall events from my childhood compared to others	54	25

Resources

Sources of Scientific Data

The facts, figures, and recommendations in this book are based on thousands of research studies conducted over the last century. But many of the extant findings reported in this book come from two studies that my colleagues and I did with funding from the National Institute of Mental Health.

- One study followed children with ADHD into adulthood. This research told us a lot about how often ADHD persists past childhood and how it changes (or stays the same) when kids with the disorder grow up.

- The other study looked at adults who had referred themselves to our clinic and ended up diagnosed with ADHD. We compared them with two other groups of adults: a group of patients being treated for other disorders but not ADHD, and a group of adults in the general population (who had not been diagnosed with any psychiatric disorder). This study gave us a much more detailed understanding of what ADHD consists of and the unique challenges it poses for adults.

You can read more about both of these studies (and many others) in this book:

Barkley, R. A., Murphy, K. R., & Fischer, M. (2008). *ADHD in adults: What the science says.* New York: Guilford Press.
- Here you'll find a lot of charts and graphs that show the data we came up with. In this book the follow-up study of children into adulthood (called a *longitudinal study*) is referred to as the "Milwaukee study." The study comparing three different groups of adults is referred to as the "UMASS study." You can also read a lot more details on specific aspects of adult ADHD if you're interested in one particular area. The list of references at the back of this book will also lead you to even further sources of information. You can order the book from The Guilford Press (*www.guilford.com*) or look for it at your local bookstore or library.

Additional Reading

The following books can give you additional insight into and advice for living with adult ADHD. Please note that much of what you'll read in them is based on clinical experience instead of research studies, but I've found that each of these books has something valuable to offer:

Adler, L., & Florence, M. (2007). *Scattered minds: Hope and help for adults with attention deficit hyperactivity disorder.* New York: G. P. Putnam's Sons.
  • A concise, clear introduction to adult ADHD written by the director of the Adult ADHD Program at the New York University School of Medicine.

American Psychiatric Association. (2013). *Diagnostic and statistical manual of mental disorders* (5th ed.). Arlington, VA: Author.
  • You can find the DSM at most libraries if you're interested in reading about the diagnostic criteria for ADHD or other disorders.

Barkley, R. A. (1994). *ADHD in adults* [videotape]. New York: Guilford Press.
  • If reading is difficult for you, watching a tape might be ideal.

Barkley, R. A. (2012). *Executive functions: What they are, how they work, and why they evolved.* New York: Guilford Press.
  • The book where I present the most recent version of my theory of executive functioning, described in Step Two.

Barkley, R. A. (2015). *Attention-deficit hyperactivity disorder: A handbook for diagnosis and treatment* (4th ed.). New York: Guilford Press.
  • Written for professionals, but if you want the comprehensive manual to refer to, this is it.

Barkley, R. A. (2017). *When an adult you love has ADHD: Professional advice for parents, partners, and siblings.* Washington, DC: APA LifeTools.
  • The first and only book to date to address the audience of parents, partners, and siblings of adults who have ADHD. A guide to understanding adult ADHD and assisting your loved one with its various problems.

Boissiere, P. (2018). *Thriving with adult ADHD: Skills to strengthen executive functioning.* San Antonio, TX: Althea Press.
  • Provides a variety of relatively simple life hacks for coping with the executive functioning deficits linked to adult ADHD.

Bramer, J. S. (1996). *Succeeding in college with attention deficit hyperactivity disorders: Issues and strategies for students, counselors, and educators.* Plantation, FL: Specialty Press. Call the ADD WareHouse at 800-233-9273 to order.
  • A valuable resource if you're in or going back to college.

Brown, T. E. (2006). *Attention deficit disorder: The unfocused mind in children and adults.* New Haven, CT: Yale University Press.
  • A fine summation of the executive deficits and other cognitive problems associated with ADHD.

CHADD. (2000). *The CHADD information and resource guide to AD/HD.* Landover, MD: Author. Go to CHADD.org or Call CHADD at 301-306-7070 to order.
- This organization dedicated to supporting children and adults with ADHD stays up on all the latest resources, listed here.

Evans, N. J., Brodo, E. M., Brown, K. R., & Wilke, A. K. (2017). *Disability in higher education: A social justice approach.* Hoboken, NJ: Jossey-Bass.

Gordon, M., & Keiser, S. (Eds.). (2000). *Accommodations in higher education under the Americans with Disabilities Act: A no-nonsense guide for clinicians, educators, administrators, and lawyers.* New York: GSI and Guilford Press.

Hallowell, E. M., & Ratey, J. J. (2005). *Delivered from distraction: Getting the most out of life with attention deficit disorder.* New York: Ballantine Books.

Hallowell, E. M., & Ratey, J. J. (2011). *Driven to distraction* (2nd ed.). New York: Pantheon.
- Very readable books by authors who have ADHD and who stress a "strength-based," positive approach to living with the disorder.

Kelly, K., & Ramundo, P. (2006). *You mean I'm not lazy, stupid, or crazy? The classic self-help book for adults with attention deficit disorder.* New York: Scribner Books.
- One of the earliest books published on adult ADHD and its symptoms. Although a bit dated now it still contains useful insights into the disorder and helpful tips for coping with its various deficits.

Kohlberg, J., & Nadeau, K. (2016). *ADD-friendly ways to organize your life.* New York: Routledge.
- Contains excellent suggestions for improving the organizational and other executive function deficits in daily life often seen in ADHD (formerly ADD).

Levrini, A., & Prevatt, F. (2012). *Succeeding with adult ADHD: Daily strategies to help you achieve your goals and manage your life.* Washington, DC: APA LifeTools.
- How to address the organizational, motivational, and time management problems associated with ADHD in adults.

Nadeau, K. G. (2007). *Survival guide for college students with ADD or LD* (2nd ed.). Washington, DC: Magination Press. Call the ADD WareHouse at 800-233-9273 to order.
- If you're a young adult in college or an older adult going back, you'll find worthy assistance here.

Nadeau, K. G. (2015). *The ADHD guide to career success* (2nd ed.). New York: Routledge.
- Provides some sage advice on accommodations to seek in the workplace and how to decide on the best employment settings that may better match with your ADHD symptoms as well as aptitudes.

Nadeau, K. G., & Quinn, P. (2002). *Understanding women with AD/HD.* Silver Spring, MD: Advantage.
- A good resource for women with ADHD.

Orlov, M. (2010). *The ADHD effect on marriage: Understand and rebuild your relationship in six steps.* Plantation, FL: Specialty Press.
- One of the few books addressing the issues related to the impact of adult ADHD on marriage and what to do to improve your relationship.

Orlov, M., & Kohlenberg, N. (2014). *The couples guide to thriving with ADHD*. Plantation, FL: Specialty Press.
- An informative guide to strategies couples can utilize when one or both have adult ADHD.

Pera, G. (2008). *Is it you, me, or adult A.D.D.?* San Francisco: 1201 Alarm Press.
- Meant for the spouses or partners of adults with ADHD, this book is friendly and full of helpful anecdotes and examples.

Ramsay, J. R. (2012). *Nonmedication treatments for adult ADHD: Evaluating impact on daily functioning and well-being*. Washington, DC: American Psychological Association.
- Although intended for professionals, this book can be informative for the educated adult with ADHD who wants a summation of the latest research findings on the various psychological treatments available for adult ADHD.

Ramsay, J. R., & Rostain, A. L. (2014). *The adult ADHD tool kit*. New York: Routledge.
- An excellent book for assisting with the time management, planning, motivational, and other executive deficits associated with ADHD in adults.

Ramsay, J. R., & Rostain, A. L. (2014). *Cognitive behavioral therapy for adult ADHD: An integrative psychosocial and medical approach*. New York: Routledge.
- A professional book providing a detailed account of how to conduct CBT for adult ADHD that focuses on the executive function deficits and other problems associated with the disorder.

Sarkis, S. M. (2006). *10 simple solutions to adult ADD: How to overcome distraction and accomplish your goals*. Oakland, CA: New Harbinger.
- Though a bit dated now, many of these suggestions are still worth considering in solving some of the problems in everyday life that exist with ADHD (ADD).

Sarkis, S. M., & Klein, K. (2009). *ADD and your money: A guide to personal finance for adults with attention-deficit disorder*. Oakland, CA: New Harbinger.
- This is a richly detailed book of advice on how to manage finances if you are an adult with ADHD and to date is the only book focusing solely on this topic.

Sarkis, S., & Tuckman, A. (2015). *Natural relief for adult ADHD: Complementary strategies for increasing focus, attention, and motivation with or without medication*. Oakland, CA: New Harbinger.
- A fine review for getting acquainted with the various alternative treatments for ADHD, many of which are popular although they lack scientific evidence for their effectiveness.

Solanto, M. V. (2013). *Cognitive-behavioral therapy for adult ADHD: Targeting executive dysfunction*. New York: Guilford Press.
- A professional clinical manual for conducting a specialized form of CBT for the executive deficits associated with adult ADHD. Provides step-by-step guidelines and clinical handouts for each of the sessions in this evidence-based training program.

Solden, S. (2012). *Women with attention deficit disorder* (2nd ed.). Nevada City, CA: Underwood Books.

    ● A pioneer in the area of books specifically for women with ADHD; audiotape also available.

Solden, S., & Frank, M. (2019). *A radical guide for women with ADHD: Embrace neurodiversity, live boldly, and break through barriers.* Oakland, CA: New Harbinger.

    ● An inspiring book for women with ADHD on how to pursue constructive change, positive thinking, and their full potential despite having ADHD.

Surman, C., & Bilkey, T. (2014). *Fast minds: How to thrive if you have ADHD (or think you might).* New York: Berkley Publishing/Penguin Random House.

    ● A fine introduction to adult ADHD with clear, effective solutions for managing it.

Tuckman, A. (2009). *More attention, less deficit: Success strategies for adults with ADHD.* Plantation, FL: Specialty Press.

    ● A fine description of ADHD and especially the numerous ways that adults with the disorder can deal with it.

Tuckman, A. (2012). *Understand your brain, get more done: The ADHD executive functions workbook.* Plantation, Fl: Specialty Press.

    ● An informative guide to various methods for dealing with deficits in executive functioning associated with adult ADHD.

Tuckman, A. (2019). *ADHD after dark: Better sex life, better relationship.* New York: Routledge.

    ● The first book to address the topic of adult ADHD and sexual behavior in intimate relationships.

Young, J. (2007). *ADHD grown up: A guide to adolescent and adult ADHD.* New York: Norton.

    ● A fine but somewhat dated resource for both professionals and people with adult ADHD.

Wilder, J. (2017). *Help for women with ADHD: My simple strategies for conquering chaos.* New York: CreateSpace Independent Publishing.

    ● Provides a wide variety of easy-to-follow recommendations for dealing with time management and organization.

Zylowska, L., & Mitchell, J. T. (2021). *Mindfulness for adult ADHD: A clinician's guide.* New York: Guilford Press.

    ● An excellent clinical manual not only summarizing the research on the use of this treatment with adults with ADHD but, better yet, providing step-by-step clinical instructions on how to implement their approach to managing ADHD in adults.

Zylowska, L., & Siegel, D. (2012). *The mindfulness prescription for adult ADHD.* Durban, South Africa: Trumpeter Publishing.

  ● The first book to set forth the use of secular mindfulness meditation for use with adults who have ADHD. Although there wasn't much evidence supporting its effectiveness when the book was published, subsequent research has suggested some promise for this approach in addressing some of the problems linked to adult ADHD. For a more current version, see the preceding book by Zylowska and Mitchell.

Rating Scales

The following scales are tools for clinicians. Each scale comes with a limited photocopy license, which allows purchasers to reproduce the forms and score sheets and yields considerable cost savings over other available scales. The large format and sturdy wire binding facilitate photocopying.

Barkley, R. A. (2011). *Barkley Adult ADHD Rating Scale–IV (BAARS-IV).* New York: Guilford Press.

  ● The Barkley Adult ADHD Rating Scale–IV (BAARS-IV) offers an essential tool for assessing current ADHD symptoms and domains of impairment as well as recollections of childhood symptoms.

Barkley, R. A. (2011). *Barkley Deficits in Executive Functioning Scale (BDEFS for Adults).* New York: Guilford Press.

  ● The Barkley Deficits in Executive Functioning Scale (BDEFS) is an empirically based tool for evaluating dimensions of adult executive functioning in daily life.

Barkley, R. A. (2011). *Barkley Functional Impairment Scale (BFIS for Adults).* New York: Guilford Press.

  ● The Barkley Functional Impairment Scale (BFIS) is the first empirically based, norm-referenced tool designed to evaluate possible impairment in 15 major domains of psychosocial functioning in adults. Clinicians must assess functional impairment before diagnosing a mental disorder or evaluating a disability claim.

Websites

General/Comprehensive Sites

ADDitude Magazine
www.additudemag.com
  ● A wealth of help for adults, from workplace resources and legal rights to household tips, travel advice, and health recommendations for adults with ADHD.

Attention Deficit Disorder Association (ADDA)
www.add.org
  ● International nonprofit organization devoted to adult ADHD. Numerous resources, links, support groups, and products.

Russell A. Barkley, PhD
www.russellbarkley.org

Canadian ADHD Resource Alliance (CADDRA)
www.caddra.ca
- Members are physicians, but there's lots of information for people who have ADHD—children, adolescents, and adults.

Centre for ADHD Awareness, Canada (CADDAC)
www.caddac.ca
- A nonprofit advocacy organization dedicated to education and advocacy for people with ADHD.

Children and Adults with Attention-Deficit Hyperactivity Disorder (CHADD)
www.chadd.org
- The largest and oldest nonprofit organization in the United States dedicated to helping people with ADHD. Many resources, links, and support groups for adults and adolescents as well as children.

Learning Disabilities Association of America (LDA)
www.ldaamerica.org
- Help for adults with learning disabilities, from screening and evaluation through accommodations for the GED and more.

National Attention Deficit Disorder Information and Support Service (ADDISS)
www.addiss.co.uk
- UK nonprofit organization whose website offers lots of resources and information and a link to the Adult ADHD Support Network.

National Institute of Mental Health (NIMH)
www.nimh.nih.gov
- Check here for updates on the latest research.

Sources for Books, Other Reading Materials, and Products

ADD WareHouse
www.addwarehouse.com
- A great online store for books, newsletters, DVDs, and products like timers.

Specific Populations

ADHD and Marriage
www.adhdmarriage.com
- A blog and forum operated by Ned Hallowell, author of *Driven to Distraction* and *Delivered from Distraction,* and Melissa Orlov specifically on how ADHD affects marital relationships.

ADHD Roller Coaster with Gina Pera: All about Adult ADHD—Especially Relationships

www.adhdrollercoaster.org

● A blog by Gina Pera, with links to current findings on the disorder and also information on being the partner of someone with ADHD.

Coaches and Coaching

ADD Coach Academy: *www.addca.com*
ADHD Coaches Organization: *www.adhdcoaches.org*
International Coaching Federation: *www.coachfederation.org*

How to Find Adult ADHD Professionals and Clinics

You can always go online and search for ADHD professionals or specialists in your city or state. You can also specifically search *www.chadd.org* and *www.additudemag.com* for ADHD professionals in your area. Or check out the *www.chadd.org* website to see if they have a chapter near your city. If so, call that chapter president and ask for recommendations on professionals. They will be very familiar with services in the area that their members will have used for their own ADHD or that of their loved ones.

Index